An Atlas of
OSTEOPOROSIS

An Atlas of
OSTEOPOROSIS
Third Edition

John C Stevenson FRCP FESC MFSEM
Consultant Physician and Reader
National Heart and Lung Institute
Imperial College London
Royal Brompton Hospital
London, UK

Michael S Marsh MD MRCOG
Consultant in Obstetrics and Gynaecology
King's College Hospital
Senior Lecturer
Guy's, King's and St Thomas' School of Medicine
London, UK

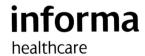

informa
healthcare

First published in the United Kingdom in 2008 by Informa Healthcare, Telephone House, 69-77 Paul Street, London EC2A 4LQ. Informa Healthcare is a trading division of Informa UK Ltd. Registered Office: 37/41 Mortimer Street, London W1T 3JH. Registered in England and Wales number 1072954.

Tel: +44 (0)20 7017 5000
Fax: +44 (0)20 7017 6699
Website: www.informahealthcare.com

A CIP record for this book is available from the British Library.
Library of Congress Cataloging-in-Publication Data

Data available on application

ISBN-10: 0 415 40429 0
ISBN-13: 978 0 415 40429 7

Distributed in North and South America by
Taylor & Francis
6000 Broken Sound Parkway, NW, (Suite 300)
Boca Raton, FL 33487, USA

Within Continental USA
Tel: 1 (800) 272 7737; Fax: 1 (800) 374 3401
Outside Continental USA
Tel: (561) 994 0555; Fax: (561) 361 6018
Email: orders@crcpress.com

Distributed in the rest of the world by
Thomson Publishing Services
Cheriton House
North Way
Andover, Hampshire SP10 5BE, UK
Tel: +44 (0)1264 332424
Email: tps.tandfsalesorder@thomson.com

Composition by Exeter Premedia Services Private Ltd., Chennai, India
Printed and bound in India by Replika Press Pvt. Ltd.

Contents

Foreword

Over the last several years, many volumes have appeared on the subject of osteoporosis. Most of these are multi-authored books with a high degree of scientific accuracy, but the usual heterogeneity in writing style. In this, the third edition of An Atlas of Osteoporosis, Drs Stevenson and Marsh have produced an exciting volume that provides cogent, up-to-date evaluation of the pathophysiology, prevention and treatment of osteoporosis. The large number of figures and diagrams render this a novel volume. This unique approach to osteoporosis provides a valuable resource for physicians who practice in the field as well as for those who see patients with osteoporosis only occasionally. It will be particularly useful for young physicians as they enter their career. Written in a readable style throughout, the many illustrations enhance the text, fulfilling the old adage, 'a picture is worth a thousand words'. Of particular importance are the images surrounding the techniques of bone densitometry, which demonstrate not only the techniques, but the output from the techniques. This provides an introduction for the practicing physician to the technology which has become of increasing clinical importance. Osteoporosis is defined as a disease of low bone density which is recognised as a major risk factor for fracture. Thus, in order to make the diagnosis, the clinician must make use of bone densitometry. However, many physicians are still wary of a test that they did not learn about in medical school or during their early training. This volume places that test in its clinical context, provides a review of a majority of the tests that are currently available and should enhance the comfort level of any practicing physician with this investigation. In situations in which the original print-outs are not provided to the practicing doctor from the densitometry unit, the illustrations here allow the clinician to provide simple explanation to the patient about the test, its meaning, its interpretation and its clinical utility.

The senior author, Dr John Stevenson, is a Reader in Medicine at Imperial College and is an international expert in the field of osteoporosis and metabolic medicine. In this volume, Dr Stevenson brings his outstanding gifts as a teacher and scientist and provides the high-quality, factual information required to make a success of this volume. He is ably supported by Dr Michael Marsh who is a Consultant Gynecologist with a thorough understanding of this disease and its importance for the Ob/Gyn community. In this third edition, they have enhanced figures, updated and revised text, and provide a detailed account of the advances that have occurred in osteoporosis in a format of particular use to clinicians. I can thoroughly recommend this book to those with both a passing and a detailed interest in this disease.

Robert Lindsay MD
Helen Hayes Hospital
West Haverstraw, New York
USA

Acknowledgements

The authors and publishers are grateful to the following for their kind permission to include some of the illustrations in this Atlas:

Mr Paul R Allen, Consultant Orthopaedic Surgeon, Princess Royal University Hospital, Orpington, Kent.

Ms Linda Banks, Superintendent Radiographer, Charing Cross Hospital, London.

Professor Alan Boyde, Professor Sheila Jones, and *Mr J. A. P. Jayasinghe,* formerly, Department of Anatomy and Developmental Biology, University College London.

Dr David Dempster and *Professor Robert Lindsay,* Regional Bone Center, Helen Hayes Hospital, West Haverstraw, New York.

Drs Kroll and Winter, Siemens AG, Berlin.

Dr Belinda Lees, Clinical Trials and Evaluation Unit, Royal Brompton Hospital, London.

Dr Flemming Melsen, University Department of Pathology, Aarhus County Hospital, Aarhus.

Dr Leif Mosekilde, University Department of Endocrinology and Metabolism, Aarhus County Hospital, Aarhus.

Eli Lilly and Company, Indianapolis, Indiana.

GE Lunar Inc., Madison, Wisconsin.

Hologic Inc., Bedford, Massachusetts.

Siemens AG, Erlangen.

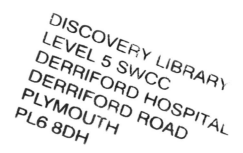
Introduction

Osteoporosis may be defined as a reduction in bone mass per unit volume such that fractures may occur with minimal trauma. It is the most common metabolic bone disease in the Western world. There are many causes, but by far the most common and most important is postmenopausal osteoporosis, which affects most women by the end of their lives.

Despite an increasing awareness of the importance of osteoporosis in some sections of the population, many women are still not sufficiently aware of the condition, do not appreciate the way in which it may affect their lives and, most importantly, do not understand that it is preventable. It is the duty of healthcare professionals to provide women with an impartial account of the current knowledge regarding osteoporosis.

CHAPTER 1

Epidemiology

AGE- AND GENDER-SPECIFIC INCIDENCE AND PREVALENCE

Osteoporosis is the most important cause of fracture in the elderly in the Western world (Figure 1.1)[1]. In the USA, at least 1.3 million fractures per year are attributable to this condition[2], of which 700 000 are vertebral fractures and 300 000 are hip fractures[3]. It is estimated that in the USA, 8 million women aged 50 or older have osteoporosis and 22 million have low bone mass[4]. By 2010, these numbers are predicted to increase to 9 million and 26 million, respectively. Estimates of fracture frequency in the UK vary, but the combined annual incidence of fracture of the vertebrae, hip, and distal forearm is approximately 200 000, of which the majority are associated with osteoporosis.

An estimated 40% of women and 13% of men aged 50 years and older will sustain an osteoporotic fracture in their lifetime[5]. Taking into account future mortality trends, these figures rise to 47% for women and 22% for men[6].

The cumulative lifetime risk of having an osteoporotic fracture is 2–4 times greater in women than in men[7]. It is difficult to calculate the economic cost of osteoporotic fractures, but it is clear that the monetary cost is high and that it is rising. In the 1980s it was estimated that the annual cost of care for patients with proximal femoral fracture alone in the USA was $8 billion[8]. More recently, direct medical expenditures for managing osteoporotic fractures were estimated to be $17 billion annually[2].

The three most common sites of osteoporotic fracture are the distal radius, the vertebral body, and the upper femur. Fractures of the distal radius invariably result from a fall onto the outstretched hand. Each year, there are approximately 40 000 such fractures in the UK[9] and 250 000 in the USA[2]; in the UK, it has been estimated that 0.5% of women over the age of 70 years will sustain this fracture each year[10]. The rate of distal forearm fracture rises sharply after the age of 50 years in women, but changes little with age in men. After the age of 65 years, the rate in women does not appear to increase further.

In England in 1985, 37 600 people aged 65 years and over sustained a fracture of the hip[11], and in the USA in 1987, there were approximately 250 000 hip fractures[2]. Whilst hip fracture is most common in elderly women, it should also be appreciated that over 9000 hip fractures per year occur in women aged between 50 and 65 years in the UK[12]. Although the increase in the age-specific rate of hip fracture that occurred in the UK between the mid-1950s and 1980[13,14] appears to have ceased more recently[13], it is likely that the proportion of elderly women in the population will continue to increase. It has been estimated that a 15% increase may be anticipated in the rate of proximal femoral fractures during the next decade simply because of aging of the population[15]. The risk of hip fracture rises approximately 1.3% per annum in women aged over 65 years[15] and at half this rate in men[16]. At age 65 years, the incidence is 1–2 per thousand for women and 0.5–1 per thousand for men. By 85 years of age, the corresponding incidences in women and men are approximately 25 and 10 per thousand, respectively[16]. The present incidence

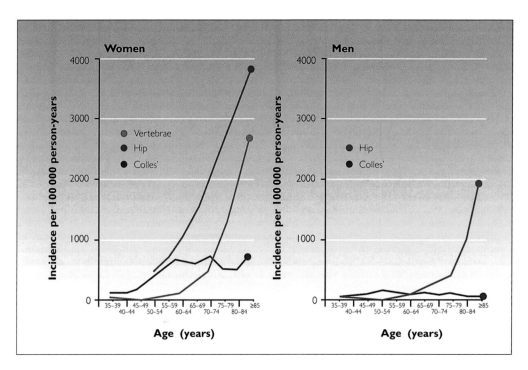

Figure 1.1 Incidence rates for the three most common osteoporotic fractures, plotted as a function of age at time of fracture. Rates are much lower in men and occur at a later age than in women. From reference 1, with permission

suggests that 15% of women over age 65 years[17] and nearly a quarter of English women living to 90 years of age[7,18] can expect to have a hip fracture.

Osteoporosis is an important cause of mortality and morbidity not only in the Western countries, because the number of elderly women is increasing worldwide, most rapidly in Asia, Latin America, the Middle East, and Africa (Figure 1.2). It has been estimated that these regions will account for more than 70% of the estimated 6.26 million fractures expected in the year 2050[8].

Hip fracture is an important cause of mortality and morbidity. Approximately 20–27% of women who sustain such a fracture die within a year[19,20]. About half of the women who have had a hip fracture will experience long-term pain and disability[15], and 20% will have severely impaired mobility a year later[19]. In the USA, which does not have a domiciliary system such as has developed in the UK, half of the survivors of a fractured hip will enter long-term nursing-home care[1].

There are few studies of the age-specific incidence of vertebral fracture as many fractures are subclinical. It has been estimated that only one-third of such events are brought to medical attention at the time of fracture[9]. The annual incidence in Rochester, Minnesota, in the 1980s was 0.5% at age 50 years, rising to 4% at age 85 years[1]. In the 1960s, Smith and Risek[21] X-rayed 2063 women in Puerto Rico and southwestern Michigan, and found a prevalence of vertebral fracture that rose with age to a maximum of approximately 20% at around 70 years of age. Data from the 1980s[17] from 134 apparently normal women showed a prevalence of wedge fracture in approximately 60% of women over age 70 years and a prevalence of crushed vertebrae of 10%. A recent prospective study[22] of 2260 women, mean age 62.2 years, recruited in 18 European centers estimated vertebral fracture by lateral spinal X-ray at baseline and 5 years later. Two hundred and forty (11%) had prevalent fractures at the baseline survey, and a further 3.8% developed incident fractures during follow-up. Vertebral fractures are at least 10 times more common in women than in men[23].

A detailed and extensive study[20] of all fractures in the town of Malmö, Sweden, during the 1950s to the 1980s showed an increasing annual age-adjusted incidence of fracture of the hip, vertebrae,

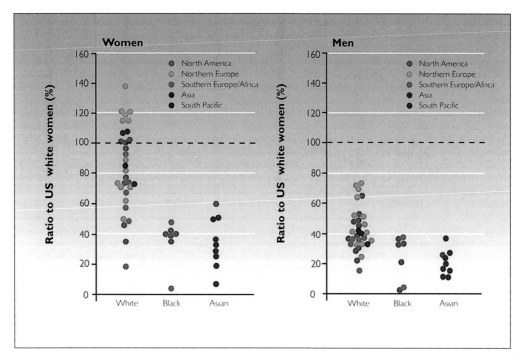

Figure 1.2 Hip fracture incidence around the world expressed as a ratio of the rates observed to those expected in the US for white women of the same age. From reference 8, with permission

and radius. This was attributed to reduced bone density resulting from declining physical activity, altered nutrition, and increased use of tobacco and/or alcohol[24]. The mortality following vertebral fracture is often overlooked, but such fractures are associated with a 20–30% mortality by 5 years[25].

RELATIONSHIP OF BONE DENSITY TO FRACTURE

Studies in which progressively increasing forces were applied to human femoral neck preparations *in vivo* have shown that the force necessary to cause fracture is linearly related to bone density[26,27]. There is little doubt that the risk of fracture is greatest in those women whose bone density is lowest.

Several prospective studies using modern methods of bone density measurement have shown a significant association between bone density and fracture risk in the female population. In the study of Hui and co-workers[28], single-photon absorptiometry (SPA) was used to measure bone density at the mid-radius in 521 white women who were followed up for an average of approximately

6.5 years. Fracture risk (excluding spinal fractures) increased with age and with decreasing radial bone density after age adjustment. The rate of increase in fracture risk with declining bone density appeared to be greater in the older age groups and in those with the lowest bone density (Figure 1.3). Overall, the risk of hip fracture alone increased 1.9 times with each g/cm decrease in radial bone mass.

Using SPA measurement at the distal and midradius, Gärdsell and colleagues[29] estimated bone density in 1076 women who were followed up for 11 years. The fracture risk was up to 7.5 times greater in the 10% of women with the lowest bone densities compared with the 10% who had the highest densities. A larger study of 9704 white women used similar methods and followed up those women who had had bone density measured in the radius and os calcis. An increased risk of hip, humeral shaft, and wrist fractures was found in those with the lowest bone densities[30,31]. Although there are correlations between bone density in the radius with those in the spine (Figure 1.4) and hip[32,33], the risk of hip fracture is more strongly associated with the bone density in

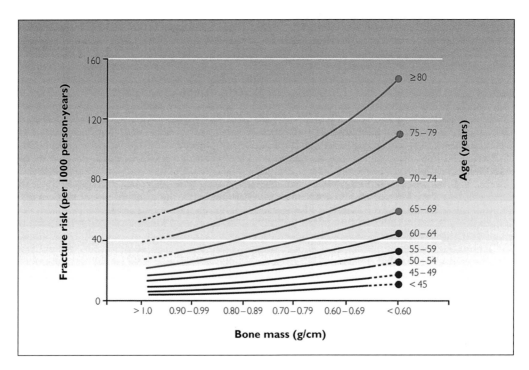

Figure 1.3 Relationship of bone density to fracture at different ages allows prediction of future fracture risk. From reference 28, with permission

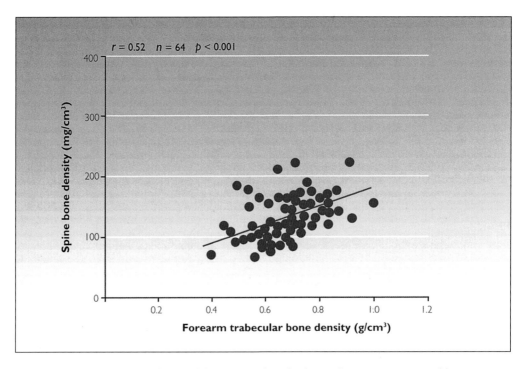

Figure 1.4 Correlation between vertebral and forearm trabecular bone density as measured by quantitative computed tomography (QCT). The relationship is highly significant, but not predictive. From reference 32, with permission

the proximal femur than in the radius[34,35]. Similarly, vertebral bone density is likely to be the best predictor of spinal fracture[36,37]. The relationship between fracture risk and bone density measured

directly at the hip and spine is stronger than that of bone density measured at peripheral sites[38].

Hip geometry may be an additional factor in fracture risk. A study[39] of hip axis length showed that this measurement was greater in women with osteoporotic fracture than in those without, suggesting that this may be a predictor of fracture independent of bone mineral density (BMD). More recent studies suggest that measurements of hip geometry may be combined with BMD to improve the prediction of fracture risk[40,41]. Further development of the measurement software and more data are required before such methods can be used in the clinical setting.

The relationship of BMD to fracture risk has been questioned by some authors. Several studies[35,42–44] have measured bone mineral density using dual-photon absorptiometry in the contralateral hip of women who had recently had a hip fracture and compared the results with age-matched controls. In all of these, and in the majority of similar but less well-conducted studies, the mean bone mineral density in women who had fractures was less than that in the controls. However, differences in the distributions of bone mineral density showed considerable overlap between the fracture and control groups. This has been interpreted by some authors to indicate that bone mineral density measurement at these sites is a poor predictor of fracture risk[18]. However, such a conclusion cannot be drawn from these data because the absence of fracture in women in the control group does not imply that they are not at risk of fracture in the future. Bone mineral density measurements are not intended to be a diagnostic test for fracture[45]. Serum cholesterol levels do not discriminate between subjects with or without coronary artery disease[46] but, as with bone mineral density measurements, can predict adverse health outcomes[47].

In summary, measurement of bone mineral density at the lumbar spine and proximal femur by dual-energy X-ray absorptiometry is currently the most appropriate way of measuring bone density to predict the risk of fracture in postmenopausal women[48]. In postmenopausal white women, the relative risk of fracture is increased by a factor of 1.5–3 for each decrease of 1.0 in the T score, depending on the site measured[49–51].

RELATIONSHIP OF FALLS TO FRACTURE

Although bone mineral density is closely associated with the risk of fracture, it does not account for all of the variation in fracture rate in the population. Age appears to be an important factor that is independent of bone mineral density. Thus, for any given bone mineral density, the fracture rate increases with age[28,52]. The relative risk increases by a factor of 2–3 per decade after the age of 28[53].

It is likely that the increased rate of falls known to occur with advancing age[54] is mainly responsible for this association. One report has shown that perimenopausal women fall more than age-matched men[55], and an increase in the rate of falls around the time of the menopause may be responsible for the sharp increase in the incidence of distal forearm fracture seen in women, but not men, at the age of 50 years[16]. Neuromuscular and visual impairment are predictors of hip fracture in elderly mobile women. A slower gait, poor heel-to-toe walking, and reduced visual acuity have been reported to be independent predictors of hip fracture in a French study of 7575 women over 75 years of age[56]. A tendency to fall in an individual is likely to persist, and may explain why the most important risk factor for fracture, independent of bone mineral density, is a previous fragility fracture. Such a fracture increases the risk of future fractures by as much as a factor of 8. The risk is highest in the first year or two after the initial fracture[57].

It has been suggested that the relative roles of falls and reduced bone mineral density as contributors to the risk of fracture are different for the three most common osteoporotic fracture types[58]. Fractures of the distal radius may be more influenced by the rate of falls than by low bone mineral density, whereas the rate of fracture of the vertebral body, greatest in an older population, may be mainly related to low bone mineral density. The rate of distal forearm fracture does not appear to increase significantly in women over 65 years old, whereas the rate of femoral neck fracture increases steadily with age as the rate of falls rises and bone mineral density declines. The vast majority of femoral fractures in the elderly are caused by simple falls on a level surface rather than more violent trauma[9]. It has been demonstrated that fractures of the femoral neck are more likely to occur in those who fall and have insufficient dexterity to use their hands to break their descent, and thus fall directly onto their hip[59].

Age and bone density can be combined to estimate the risk of any fragility fracture during the subsequent 5 or 10 years. For example, the 10-year risk of fragility fracture in a postmenopausal woman with a T score of −2.5 or less with no other risk factors is less than 5% at age 50 but more than 20% at age 65. The risk increases more with the addition of other risk factors, especially a previous fragility fracture[60].

REFERENCES

1. Riggs BL, Melton LJ. Involutional osteoporosis. N Engl J Med 1986; 314: 1676–86.

2. Melton LJ IIIrd. Etiology, diagnosis and management. In: Riggs B, Melton LI, eds. Epidemiology of Fractures. New York: Raven Press, 1988: 133–54.

3. National Osteoporosis Foundation. Disease statistics. http://www.nof.org/osteoporosis/stats.htm.

4. National Osteoporosis Foundation. America's Bone Health: The State of Osteoporosis and Low Bone Mass in Our Nation. Washington, DC: National Osteoporosis Foundation, 2002.

5. Melton LJ 3rd, Chrischilles EA, Cooper C, Lane AW, Riggs BL. Perspective. How many women have osteoporosis? J Bone Miner Res 1992; 7: 1005–10.

6. Kanis JA, Johnell O, Oden A et al. Long-term risk of osteoporotic fracture in Malmo. Osteoporosis Int 2000; 11: 669–74.

7. Consensus conference: Osteoporosis. JAMA 1984; 252: 99–802.

8. Melton LJ IIIrd. Hip fractures: a worldwide problem today and tomorrow. Bone 1993; 14 (Suppl 1): S1–8.

9. Grimley Evans J. The significance of osteoporosis. In: Smith R, ed. Osteoporosis. London: Royal College of Physicians, 1990: 1–8.

10. Alffram PS, Bauer G. Epidemiology of fractures of the forearm. J Bone Joint Surg 1962; 44 (A): 105–14.

11. Office of Population Censuses and Surveys. Hospital Inpatient Enquiry, 1985. London: HMSO, 1987.

12. Stevenson JC. HRT, osteoporosis and regulatory authorities. Quis custodiat ipsos custodies? Hum Reprod 2006; 21: 1668–71.

13. Spector TD, Cooper C, Fenton Lewis A. Trends in admissions for hip fracture in England and Wales. BMJ 1990; 300: 173–4.

14. Boyce WJ, Vessey MP. Rising incidence of fracture of the proximal femur. Lancet 1985; 1: 150–1.

15. Lindsay R, Hart DM. The minimum effective dose of estrogen for prevention of postmenopausal bone loss. Obstet Gynecol 1984; 63: 759–63.

16. Grimley Evans J, Prudham D, Wandles I. A prospective study of fractured proximal femur: Incidence and outcome. Public Health (London) 1979; 93: 235–41.

17. Nordin BEC, Crilly RG, Smith DA. Osteoporosis. In: Nordin B, ed. Metabolic Bone and Stone Disease. Edinburgh: Churchill Livingstone, 1984: 1–70.

18. Law MR, Wald NJ, Meade TW. Strategies for prevention of osteoporosis and hip fracture. BMJ 1991; 303: 453–9.

19. Miller CW. Survival and ambulation following hip fractures. J Bone Joint Surg 1978; 60 (A): 930–4.

20. NIH Consensus Development Panel on Osteoporosis Prevention, Diagnosis, and Therapy. Osteoporosis prevention, diagnosis and therapy. JAMA 2001; 285: 320–3.

21. Smith RW, Risek J. Epidemiological studies of osteoporosis in women of Puerto Rico and southwestern Michigan. Clin Orthop 1962; 45: 31–48.

22. O'Neill TW, Cockerill W, Matthis C et al. Back pain, disability, and radiographic vertebral fracture in European women: a prospective study. Osteoporos Int 2004; 15: 760–5.

23. Lindsay R. Pathogenesis, detection and prevention of postmenopausal osteoporosis. In: Studd J, Whitehead M, eds. The Menopause. Oxford: Blackwell Scientific Publications, 1988: 156–67.

24. Obrant K, Bengnér U, Johnell O et al. Increasing age-adjusted risk of fragility fractures: a sign of increasing osteoporosis in successive generations? Calcif Tissue Int 1989; 44: 157–67.

25. Kanis JA, Johnell O, Oden A et al. Epidemiology of osteoporosis and fracture in men. Calcif Tissue Int 2004; 75: 90–9.

26. Leichter I, Margulies JY, Weinreb A et al. The relationship between bone density, mineral content, and mechanical strength in the femoral neck. Clin Orthop 1982; 163: 272–81.

27. Dalen N, Hellstrom L-G, Jacobson B. Bone mineral content and mechanical strength of the femoral neck. Acta Orthop Scand 1976; 47: 503–8.

28. Hui SL, Slemenda CW, Johnson CC Jr. Age and bone mass as predictors of fracture in a prospective study. J Clin Invest 1988; 81: 1804–9.

29. Gardsell P, Johnell O, Nilsson BE. Predicting fractures in women using forearm bone densitometry. Calcif Tissue Int 1989; 44: 355–61.

30. Browner WS, Cummings SR, Genat HK. Bone mineral density and fractures of the wrist and humerus in elderly women: a prospective study. J Bone Miner Res 1989; 4 (Suppl): S171.

31. Cummings SR, Black DM, Nevitt MC et al. Appendicular bone density and age predict hip fractures in women. JAMA 1990; 263: 665–8.

32. Stevenson JC, Banks LM, Spinks TJ et al. Regional and total skeletal measurements in the early postmenopause. J Clin Invest 1987; 80: 258–62.

33. Ott SM, Kilcoyne RF, Chesnut CH IIIrd. Ability of four different techniques of measuring bone mass to diagnose vertebral fractures in postmenopausal women. J Bone Miner Res 1987; 2: 201–10.

34. Mazess RB, Barden H, Ettinger M et al. Bone density of the radius, spine, and proximal femur in osteopororsis. J Bone Miner Res 1988; 3: 13–18.

35. Riggs BL, Wahner HW, Seeman E et al. Changes in bone mineral density of the proximal femur and spine with aging. Differences between the postmenopausal and senile osteoporosis syndromes. J Clin Invest 1982; 70: 716–23.

36. Nordin BEC, Wishart JM, Horowitz M et al. The relation between forearm and vertebral mineral density and fractures in postmenopausal women. Bone Miner 1988; 5: 21–33.

37. Eastell R, Wahner HW, O'Fallon WM et al. Unequal decrease in bone density of lumbar spine and ultradistal radius in Colles' and vertebral fracture syndromes. J Clin Invest 1989; 83: 168–74.

38. Marshall D, Johnell O, Wedel H. Meta-analysis of how well measures of bone mineral density predict occurrence of osteoporotic fractures. BMJ 1996; 312: 1254–9.

39. Boonen S, Koutri R, Dequeker J et al. Measurement of femoral geometry in type I and type II osteoporosis: differences in hip axis length consistent with heterogeneity in the pathogenesis of osteoporotic fractures. J Bone Miner Res 1995; 10: 1908–12.

40. El-Kaissi S, Pasco JA, Henry MJ et al. Femoral neck geometry and hip fracture risk: the Geelong osteoporosis study. Osteoporos Int 2005; 16: 1299–303.

41. Crabtree NJ, Kroger H, Martin A et al. Improving risk assessment: hip geometry, bone mineral distribution and bone strength in hip fracture cases and controls. The EPOS study. European Prospective Osteoporosis International 2002; 13: 48–54.

42. Chevalley T, Rizzoli R, Nydegger V et al. Preferential low bone mineral density of the femoral neck in patients with a recent fracture of the proximal femur. Osteoporos Int 1991; 1: 147–54.

43. Eriksson SAV, Wilde TL. Bone mass in women with hip fracture. Orthop Scand 1988; 59: 19–23.

44. Bohr H, Schaadt O. Bone mineral content of femoral bone and the lumbar spine measured in women with fracture of the femoral neck by dual photon absorptiometry. Clin Orthop 1983; 179: 240–5.

45. Davis JW, Vogel JM, Ross PD, Wasnich RD. Disease versus etiology: the distinction should not be lost in the analysis. J Nucl Med 1989; 112: 1273–6.

46. Rose G. Sick individuals and sick populations. Int J Epidemiol 1985; 14: 32–8.

47. Stevenson JC, Marsh MS. Preventing osteoporosis [Letter]. BMJ 1991; 303: 920–1.

48. Bates DW, Black DM, Cummings SR. Clinical use of bone densitometry: clinical applications. JAMA 2002; 288: 1898–900.

49. Johnell O, Kanis JA, Black DM et al. Associations between baseline risk factors and vertebral fracture risk in the Multiple Outcomes of Raloxifene Evaluation (MORE) Study. J Bone Miner Res 2004; 19: 764–72.

50. Cummings SR, Nevitt MC, Browner WS et al. Risk factors for hip fracture in white women. N Engl J Med 1995; 332: 767–73.

51. Schuit SC, van der Klift M, Weel AE et al. Fracture incidence and association with bone mineral density in elderly men and women: the Rotterdam Study. Bone 2004; 34: 195–202.

52. Ross PD, Wasnich RD, McClean CJ et al. A model for estimating the potential costs and savings of osteoporosis prevention strategies. Bone 1988; 9: 337–47.

53. Cauley JA, Zmuda JM, Wisniewski SR et al. Bone mineral density and prevalent vertebral fractures in men and women. Osteoporos Int 2004; 15: 32–7.

54. Cummings SR. Are patients with hip fractures more osteoporotic? Am J Med 1985; 78: 487–94.

55. Winner SJ, Morgan A, Grimley Evans J. Perimenopausal risk of falling and incidence of distal forearm fracture. BMJ 1989; 298: 1486–8.

56. Dargent-Molina P, Favier F, Grandjean H et al. Fall-related factors and risk of hip fracture: the EPIDOS prospective study. Epidémiologie de l'ostéoporose. Lancet 1996; 348: 145–9.

57. Lindsay R, Silverman SL, Cooper C et al. Risk of new vertebral fracture in the year following a fracture. JAMA 2001; 285: 320–3.

58. Kanis JA, Aaron J, Thavarajah M et al. Osteoporosis: causes and therapeutic implications. In: Smith R, ed. Osteoporosis. London: Royal College of Physicians, 1990: 45–56.

59. Nevitt MC, Cummings SR. Type of fall and risk of hip and wrist fractures: the study of osteoporotic fractures. The Study of Osteoporotic Fractures Research Group. J Am Geriatr Soc 1993; 41: 1226–34.

60. Kanis JA, Johnell O, De Laet C et al. A meta-analysis of previous fracture and subsequent fracture risk. Bone 2004; 35: 375–82.

Bone structure

CORTICAL AND TRABECULAR BONE

Bone provides the strength and rigidity of the skeleton as well as acting as a reservoir of calcium and other mineral salts. It is a highly vascular, mineralized connective tissue of cells in a fibrous organic matrix permeated by inorganic bone salts. The collagen framework varies from an almost random network to highly organized sheets or helical bundles of parallel fibers. Mature bone may be classified into two types, cortical or compact, and trabecular or cancellous.

Cortical bone is always found on the outside of bones and surrounds the trabecular bone (Figure 2.1). Approximately 80% of the skeleton is cortical bone. The architecture and amount of cortical bone at any site are related to its function at that area. Cortical bone is porous, but the ratio of solid tissue to space is considerably higher than for trabecular bone. Cortical bone is made up of a collection of cylindrical units termed Haversian systems, which run parallel to the outer surface of the bone. Each Haversian system has a central Haversian canal containing a neurovascular bundle, and each canal is surrounded by concentric lamellae of bony tissue (Figure 2.2). The lamellae are separated by small spaces termed lacunae, which are connected to each other and to the central Haversian canal by small channels called canaliculi. Osteocytes are found within the lacunae and extend cytoplasmic processes into the canaliculi. The gaps between the Haversian systems are made up of interstitial bone which consists of similar tissue elements, but in a less organized pattern. Haversian systems are separated from one another by cement lines which are strongly basophilic, have a high content of inorganic matrix, and correspond to areas of bone resorption and deposition.

Trabecular bone is found in the middle of bones such as the vertebrae, pelvis, and other flat bones, and at the ends of the long bones. It consists mainly of more fragmented systems of Haversian lamellae and lacunae covered by numerous cement lines separated by large spaces filled with bone marrow. Trabecular bone receives its blood supply from the surrounding tissues. The high surface area-to-volume ratio of trabecular bone indicates that it is far more metabolically active compared with cortical bone and has the potential to change its density more rapidly.

BONE CELLS

There are three main types of bone cells: osteoblasts, osteoclasts, and osteocytes.

Osteoblasts

These cells originate from bone marrow-derived stromal cells[3] and are responsible for the deposition of the extracellular matrix and its mineralization[4]. They are highly differentiated columnar-shaped cells (20–30 μm in diameter), usually found in a layer one cell thick, intimately apposed to areas of bone formation or remodeling (Figure 2.3). They have a cellular structure that includes extensive endoplasmic reticulum, a large Golgi complex, and other cellular characteristics, in keeping with

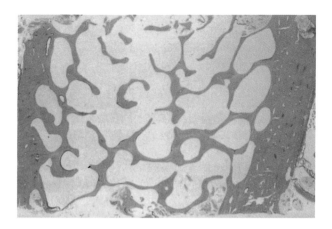

Figure 2.1 Normal iliac crest bone (Goldner's trichrome stain) showing inner and outer cortices and intervening trabecular bone. From reference 1, with permission

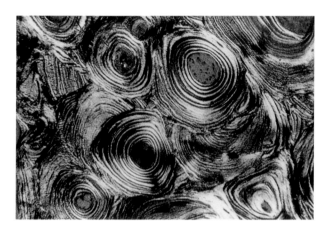

Figure 2.2 Photomicrograph of cortical bone showing concentric lamellae surrounding the central Haversian canal. From reference 2, with permission

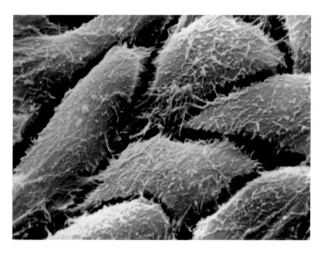

Figure 2.3 Scanning electron micrograph (SEM) of a layer or 'pavement' of osteoblasts. Courtesy of Professor Sheila Jones

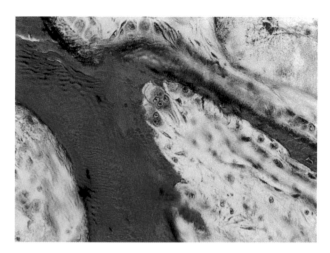

Figure 2.4 Histology showing osteoblasts on one side of a trabecular structure with multinucleated osteoclasts on the other. Osteoblasts are polarized, mononuclear, fusiform to cuboidal cells with basophilic cytoplasm. They form bone matrix (osteoid) which minerallizes in a two-phase process to mature bone. Courtesy of Dr Flemming Melsen

their role as protein-synthesizing and -secreting cells. Whereas the 'plump' osteoblasts are active in bone formation (Figure 2.4), flatter and more inactive or 'resting' osteoblasts form the lining cells on the surface of bone. These lining cells may be responsible for removing the thin layer of osteoid which coats the bone surface, thus exposing the bone for osteoclastic resorption.

Osteoclasts

Osteoclasts are responsible for the resorption of calcified bone and cartilage (Figures 2.5 and 2.6). They are derived from hemopoietic stem cells and are formed by the fusion of mononuclear cell precursors[5]. Their morphological and phagocytic characteristics are similar to other cells of the mononuclear phagocytic cell line. They are typically large (up to 200 000 μm^3) and may contain up to 100 nuclei. The cells show cellular polarity, and resorption occurs along the 'ruffled' border of the cell apposed to the bone surface. The cytoplasm adjacent to this surface is devoid of organelles, but is rich in actin filaments and other microfilament-associated proteins[6], suggesting that this area contains the source of osteoclastic bone adhesion.

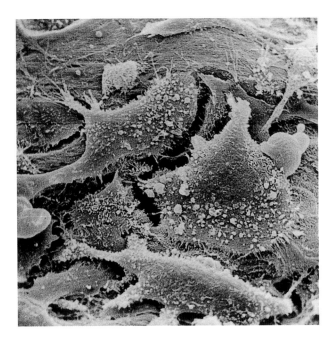

Figure 2.5 SEM of osteoclasts in *vitro*. Courtesy of Professor Alan Boyde

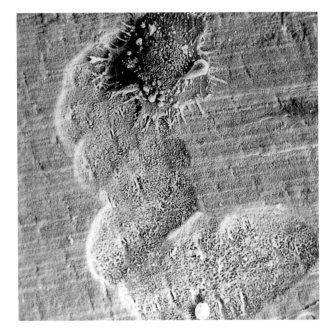

Figure 2.6 SEM showing osteoclastic resorption of bone *in vitro*. Courtesy of Professor Alan Boyde

Osteocytes

Osteocytes are osteoblasts that remain behind in lacunae (Figure 2.7) when the bone-forming surface advances. They are the result of osteoblasts 'self-entombed' by their own bone matrix-secreting activity. As they become further isolated from the bone-forming surface, their protein-synthesizing

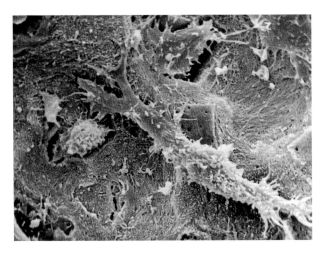

Figure 2.7 SEM of osteocytes in the bone lacunae. A 'liberated' osteocyte is seen on the surface. Courtesy of Professor Alan Boyde

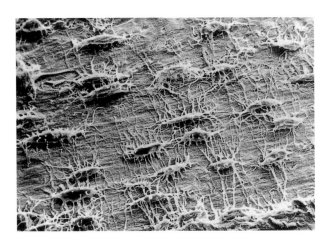

Figure 2.8 SEM of a cast to show osteocytes and their canalicular processes. Courtesy of Professor Alan Boyde

activity declines, the size of the endoplasmic reticulum and Golgi apparatus decreases, and the mitochondrial content falls. Osteocytes communicate with one another via cytoplasmic processes (Figure 2.8) that pass through the bone canaliculi. These processes may help to coordinate the response of bone to stress or deformation.

BONE PROTEINS AND MINERALS

Normal adult bone is termed lamellar bone. Each lamella is a thin plate 5–7 μm thick and made up of bone matrix consisting of protein fibers impregnated with bone salts. In each lamella, the protein fibers are largely oriented parallel to one another

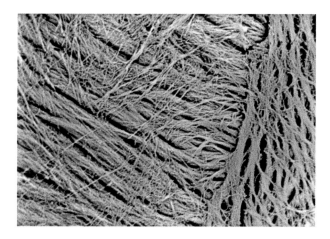

Figure 2.9 SEM of lamellar bone matrix showing the pattern of the collagen fibers. Courtesy of Professor Alan Boyde

(Figure 2.9). The organic matrix constitutes 30–40%, and mineral salts 60–70%, of the dry weight of bone. Water makes up 20% of the weight of the matrix of mature bone.

The principal organic component in bone is type I collagen, which constitutes 90–95% of the organic matrix. It is a heteropolymer of two $\alpha 1$ chains and one $\alpha 2$ chain wound together in a triple helix. The important ionic components of the bone matrix are calcium, phosphate, magnesium, carbonate, hydroxyl, fluoride, citrate, and chloride. The most important crystalline component of bone is hydroxyapatite ($Ca_{10}(PO_4)_6(OH)_2$), found as needle-shaped crystals 20–40 nm in length and 3–6 nm in breadth, generally lying with their long axes parallel to the collagen fibers. The other bone mineral ions are found in association with the surface of the hydroxyapatite crystals, or they may replace phosphate ions within the crystals.

BONE REMODELING

Bone is remodeled by osteoclasts and osteoblasts working in combination in a cycle of activity that lasts around 3–6 months. The resorption of bone by osteoclasts and its replacement by osteoblasts are normally 'coupled' together, which ensures that the processes of bone destruction and formation are more or less matched. This coupling is probably mediated by cellular messengers produced by each cell type.

In the remodeling process (Figure 2.10), the osteoclast moves to an area of bone to be remodeled and secretes lactate or hydrogen ions through its ruffled cell border onto the bone surface to create an acid environment into which proteases such as proteoglycanase and collegenase are secreted from within the cell[8]. The bone matrix is then broken down by these enzymes, perhaps with the assistance of calcium chelating ions, such as citrate, which help to solubilize minerals (Figures 2.11 and 2.12). It is possible that released proteins such as bone morphogenic proteins act as signals or 'coupling factors' for the osteoblasts. After breakdown of the bone matrix is complete, the osteoclasts disappear. Several days later, osteoblasts move to the remodelling site, first to deposit extracellular matrix, and subsequently to control its mineralization[4,9]. The chief protein secreted is type I collagen. The remodeling process occurs in both cortical (Figures 2.13 and 2.14) and trabecular (Figure 2.15) bone. Recent evidence suggests that osteoblastic activity is influenced by multiple factors including osteocrin, a recently discovered bone-active molecule, which in animals is highly expressed in cells of the osteoblast lineage. Osteocrin levels appear to correlate with osteoblast[10] and megakaryocyte activity[11].

A study of osteoid seams, resorption cavities, and bone structural units in iliac crest trabecular bone suggests that the above explanation of bone remodeling may be overly simplistic. It appears that, in some remodeling units, bone formation may start before complete resorption, bone resorption may be arrested in some cavities, and bone may be formed on quiescent bone surfaces[12]. The results of further studies are awaited.

REGULATION OF BONE CELL ACTIVITY

Bone cell activity may be regulated by local or systemic factors (Table 2.1).

Systemic factors

The three main systemic hormones that regulate calcium homeostasis (calcitonin, vitamin D, and parathyroid hormone (PTH)) all appear to have

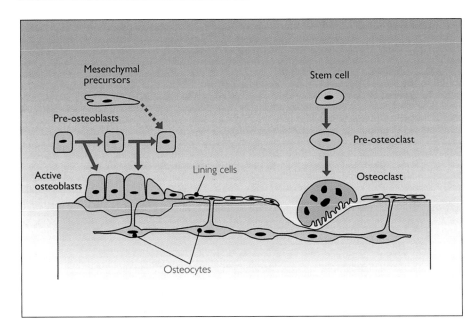

Figure 2.10 Diagrammatic representation of the developing and mature cells of bone to show the relationship between osteocytes and surface cells. From reference 7, with permission

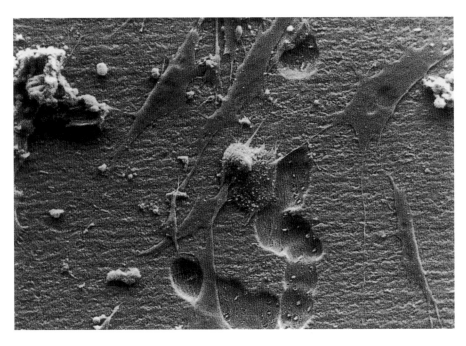

Figure 2.11 SEM from a time-lapse video of osteoclastic bone resorption showing a track of resorption pits. Courtesy of Professor Alan Boyde.

direct effects on bone cells. The principal action of calcitonin is to inhibit bone resorption. Parathyroid hormone produces changes in the shape of osteoblasts, which is thought to be indicative of increased bone resorption[13] (Figure 2.16). It is probable that 1,25-dihydroxyvitamin D_3 has effects on both osteoblasts and osteoclasts. It increases osteoblastic production of osteocalcin and alkaline phosphatase, and stimulates osteoclastic differentiation and multinucleation[14].

Estrogen has an important action in preserving bone, and estrogen hormone replacement therapy (HRT) is a proven treatment for preventing osteoporosis. Estrogen deficiency increases the rate of bone remodeling, as well as the amount of bone loss with each remodeling cycle. Animal and cell culture studies suggest that there are multiple sites of estrogen action, not only on the cells of the bone remodeling unit, but on other marrow cells. The mechanism of action is not known, but potential sites of action include effects on T cell cytokine production, effects on stromal or osteoblastic cells to alter receptor activator of nuclear factor κB ligand (RANKL) or osteoprotegerin

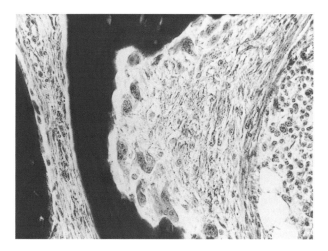

Figure 2.12 Histology from a patient with primary hyperparathyroidism showing a resorption lacuna in trabecular bone (Howship's lacuna) with multinucleated osteoclasts. Osteoclastic bone resorption includes bone matrix as well as bone mineral. The final depth of the resorption lacuna which reflects the amount of activity of the osteoclasts, is measured by counting the number of missing lamellae. Courtesy of Dr Flemming Melsen

(OPG) production, direct inhibition of differentiated osteoclasts, and effects on bone formation in response to mechanical forces initiated by osteoblasts or osteocytes[15].

Estrogen acts through two receptors, α and β. α Receptors appear to be the chief mediator of estrogen's actions on the skeleton[16]. Osteoblasts have estrogen receptors (ERs) (Figure 2.17) and express ERβ, but the actions of ERβ agonists on bone are less clear. Some reports suggest that the effects of estrogen signaling through α and β receptors are in opposition, while other studies suggest that activation of these receptors has similar effects on bone[18,19]. Functional estradiol receptors have not been identified in osteoclasts (Figure 2.18), but estrogen effects on bone may also be via an action on cells of the hematopoietic lineage, including osteoclast precursors and mature osteoclasts via cytokines and growth factors[13] which may be mediated by T cells[20]. A direct

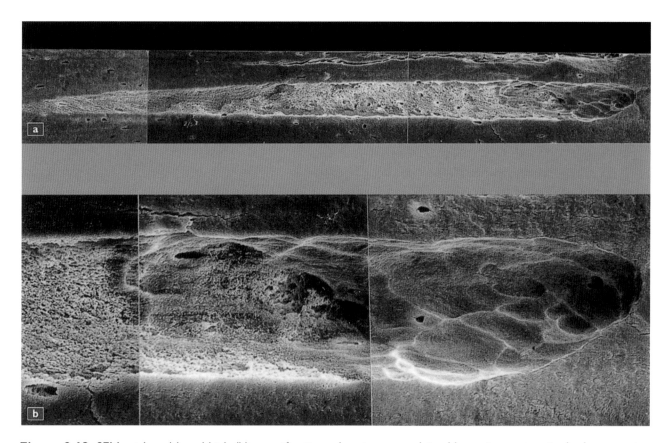

Figure 2.13 SEMs at low (a) and high (b) magnifications showing an evolving Haversian system in the bone cortex (viewed longitudinally). The cutting zone (to the right) is followed by the reversal zone and the mineralization front, with new bone then closing the canal. From reference 2, with permission

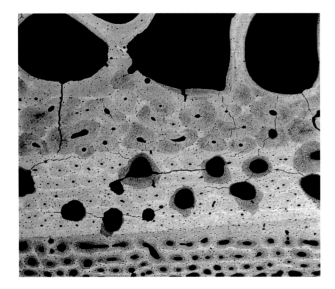

Figure 2.14 Back-scattered electron micrograph showing stages of bone remodeling. The outer (lower) cortex shows predominantly resorption and many Haversian canals whereas the inner (upper) cortex near the trabecular surface shows new bone formation closing the canals. There is a mixed pattern in the central cortical area. Courtesy of Professor Alan Boyde

effect of estrogen in accelerating osteoclast apoptosis may be due to increased transforming growth factor-β (TGF-β) production[21].

Several studies have shown that estrogens increase calcitonin secretion in both pre- and postmenopausal women[22–26], although some studies have not[27]. Calcitonin secretion has been shown to be reduced in studies of established osteoporotics compared with controls[28], but other studies have not shown this effect[29]. It is possible that the different results of calcitonin studies are due to variations in measurement techniques, including the ability of different antisera to recognize different heterogeneous molecular species, and differences in extraction techniques.

Local factors

Local factors include cytokines, growth factors, other peptides, and nitric oxide. A cytokine is a peptide produced by a cell that acts as an autocrine, paracrine, or endocrine mediator[14]. A large and increasing number of cytokines have been shown to have an effect on bone. Important cytokines include interleukin-1 (IL-1), interleukin-6 (IL-6),

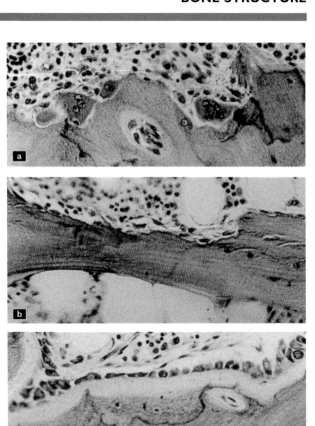
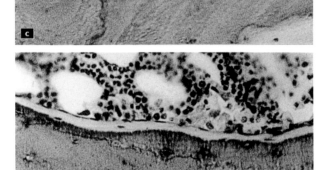
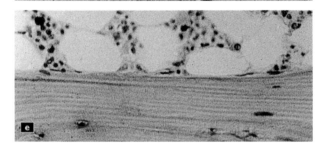

Figure 2.15 Histological biopsy sections from the iliac crest show the principal phases of the remodeling cycle in trabecular bone: resorption by osteoclasts (a); reversal, with disappearance of the osteoclasts (b); formation, with deposition of osteoid by osteoblasts (c); mineralization of the osteoid (d); and completion of the cycle (e). From reference 2, with permission

Table 2.1 Factors affecting bone resorption and formation (some assignments are tentative)

Factors	Resorption	Formation
Systemic		
PTH/PTH-related peptide	+	±
1,25-dihydroxyvitamin D$_3$	+	±
Calcitonin	−	?+
Estrogen, androgen	−	+
Glucocorticoid	+	±
Retinoid	±	±
Insulin	?	+
Growth hormone	?	+
Thyroid hormone	+	±
Local		
Prostanoid	±	+
Interleukin-1	+	±
Interleukin-4	−	?
Interleukin-6	?+	?
Colony-stimulating factor	+	−
Tumor necrosis factor	+	?
Interferon-γ	−	?
Leukemia inhibitory factor	+	?
Insulin-like growth factors I and II	?	+
Transforming growth factor-β	+	?
Epidermal growth factor	+	?
Transforming growth factor-α	±	+
Bone morphogenic protein	?	+
Platelet-derived growth factor	?	+
Fibroblast growth factor	?	?
Vasoactive intestinal peptide	+	?
Calcitonin gene-related peptide	−	?
Heparin	+	?
Miscellaneous		
Proton	+	?−
Calcium	−	+
Phosphate	+	?
Fluoride	−	+
Bisphosphonate	−	?
Antiestrogen	−	?+
Gallium nitrate	−	?
Alcohol, tobacco	?	−
Electric current	+	+
Immobilization, weightlessness	+	−
Stress, exercise	±	+

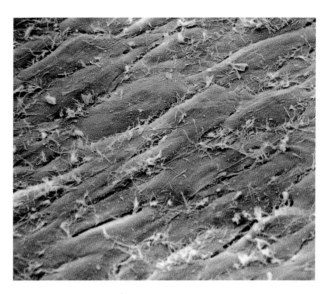

Figure 2.16 SEM of the effects of parathyroid hormone on osteoblasts. There is initial separation followed by spreading and elongation of the cells, which become multilayered. Withdrawal of parathyroid hormone leads to an increase in cell mitosis[13]. Courtesy of Professor Sheila Jones

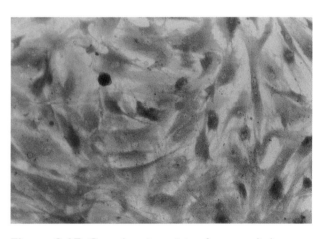

Figure 2.17 Cytoplasmic staining for estradiol receptor-related protein (p29 antigen) results in intense staining of primary human trabecular osteoblast-like cells. From reference 17, with permission

tumor necrosis factor (TNF)-α, and interferon (IFN)-γ.

IL-1 is a monocyte/macrophage product found in two forms, α and β, which appear to have similar biological activity. IL-1 stimulates some osteoblast-like cells to secrete proteinases, such as collagenase and stromelysin, which may contribute to the breakdown of connective tissue matrices[22]. The production of IL-1 after the menopause

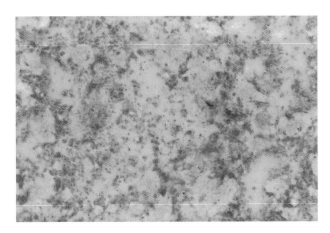

Figure 2.18 Cytoplasmic staining for estradiol receptor-related protein (p29 antigen) in human giant cell tumor imprint. Osteoclasts are clearly visible because of their lack of staining. From reference 17, with permission

is increased, and, in patients with osteoporosis, may be suppressed by estrogen therapy[29]. IL-1α, IL-1β and IL-1β mRNA are expressed significantly more in bone from osteoporotic women than from women with normal bone mineral density or postmenopausal women taking HRT[30,31].

TNF is also found in α and β forms, which are similar in activity to each other and to IL-1. Both TNF-α and IL-1 inhibit bone resorption and formation[32,33]. IL-1 and TNF-α may act in synergy and induce the production of each other as well as other cytokines.

IFN-γ inhibits IL-1- or TNF-α-induced bone resorption, but has less effect on resorption stimulated by parathyroid hormone or 1,25-dihydroxyvitamin D$_3$[34], and may be considered a potential antagonist to IL-1 and TNF-α.

Numerous growth factors that directly influence bone cell activity have been identified, and include platelet-derived growth factor (PDGF), insulin-like growth factors, and transforming growth factor (TGF)-β. PDGF stimulates bone resorption, is mitogenic for fibroblasts, and may mediate the mitogenic effects of IL-1[14]. TGF-β is produced in an inactive form which is activated by an acid environment. Estrogens may prevent bone loss by limiting osteoclastic lifespan through promotion of apoptosis mediated by TGF-β[35].

Nitric oxide (NO) has recently been found to have important effects on bone. Forms of nitric oxide synthase are expressed by bone-derived cells, and IL-1, TNF-α, and IFN-γ are potent stimulators of nitric oxide production[36]. When combined with other cytokines, IFN-γ induces nitric oxide production, which suppresses osteoclast formation and activity of mature osteoclasts. High nitric oxide concentrations inhibit cells of the osteoblast lineage, and nitric oxide production may be partly responsible for the inhibitory effects of cytokines on osteoblast proliferation. At lower nitric oxide concentrations, the effects appear to be different. Moderate induction of nitric oxide potentiates bone resorption and promotes osteoblast-like cell proliferation and function[37]. It is likely that nitric oxide is one of the molecules produced by osteoblasts that regulate osteoclast activity[38,39].

Proton secretion by the ruffled border of osteoclasts is necessary to solubilize bone mineral and degrade the organic matrix of bone. One or two protons are secreted for every Ca^{2+} liberated[40]. This secretion is mediated via an electrogenic H(+)-adenosine triphosphatase (ATPase) coupled to a chloride channel in the ruffled membrane. Antiresorptive agents such as tiludronate may partially act by inhibiting H(+)-ATPase[41]. Changes in pH may be of importance, as the regulation of bone resorption and osteoclasts is acutely sensitive to pH.

Recent studies of the molecular mechanism for the interaction between cells of the osteoblastic and osteoclastic lineages indicate that RANKL and OPG and members of the TNF-α and TNF-α receptor superfamily are important[15].

Osteoblasts produce RANKL, which activates osteoclast differentiation and maintains their function. Osteoblasts also produce and secrete OPG, which can block RANKL/RANK interactions. Bone resorption stimulators increase RANKL expression in osteoblasts, and some decrease OPG expression[42]. Recently, a monoclonal antibody against RANKL was shown to produce prolonged inhibition of bone resorption in postmenopausal women. It was also shown that RANKL levels were increased on the surface of bone marrow cells from early postmenopausal women, who are estrogen deficient[43].

However, the importance of OPG deficiency in the pathogenesis of osteoporosis has not been demonstrated, as OPG levels are not consistently different from normals in cases of osteoporosis. OPG levels increase with age, and it has been suggested that OPG production rises as a homeostatic response to limit the bone loss that occurs with an increase in other bone-resorbing factors[15,44,45].

Bone-resorbing factors can also stimulate cyclooxygenase-2 (COX-2) activity, which may amplify RANKL and OPG responses by producing prostaglandins. In summary, the RANKL/RANK interaction may represent a final common pathway for any pathogenetic factor in osteoporosis that causes increasing bone resorption[15].

Many other systemic and local factors have been shown to act directly on bone cells. For a full description, the interested reader is referred to other recent texts[15,46].

REFERENCES

1. Dempster DW, Shane E. Principles and Practice of Endocrinology and Metabolism. Philadelphia: JB Lippincott Co. 1990: 475–80.

2. Coe F, Farus MJ, eds. Disorders of Bone and Mineral Metabolism. New York: Raven Press, 1992.

3. Owen M, Ashton B. Osteogenic differentiation of different skeletal cell populations. In: Ali S, ed. Cell Mediated Calcification and Matrix Vesicles. Amsterdam: Elsevier, 1986: 279–84.

4. Anderson HC. Matrix vesicle calcification: review and update. Bone Miner Res 1985; 3: 109–49.

5. Schneider GB, Relfson M, Nicolas J. Pluripotential hemopoietic stem cells give rise to osteoclasts. Am J Anat 1986; 177: 505–12.

6. Marchisio PC, Cirillo D, Naldini L et al. Cell substratum interaction of cultured avian osteoclasts is mediated by specific adhesion structures. J Cell Biol 1984; 99: 1696–705.

7. Stevenson JC, Lindsay RL. Osteoporosis. London: Chapman & Hall, 1998.

8. Vaes G. Cellular biology and biochemical mechanisms of bone resorption. Clin Orthop 1988; 231: 239–71.

9. Russell RGG, Caswell AM, Hearn PR et al. Calcium in mineralised tissues and pathological calcification. Br Med Bull 1986; 42: 435–46.

10. Bord S, Ireland DC, Moffatt P et al. Characterization of osteocrin expression in human bone. J Histochem Cytochem 2005; 53: 1181–7.

11. Bord S, Frith E, Ireland DC et al. Megakaryocytes modulate osteoblast synthesis of type-I collagen, osteoprotegerin, and RANKL. Bone 2005; 36: 812–19.

12. Yamaguchi K, Croucher PI, Compston JE. Comparison between the lengths of individual osteoid seams and resorption cavities in human iliac crest cancellous bone. Bone Miner 1993; 23: 27–33.

13. Jones SJ, Boyd A. Experimental study of changes in osteoblastic shape induced by calcitonin and parathyroid extract in an organ culture system. Cell Tissue Res 1976; 169: 449–55.

14. Russell RGG. Bone cell biology: the role of cytokines and other mediators. In: Smith R, ed. Osteoporosis. London: Royal College of Physicians, 1990; 9–33.

15. Raisz LG. Pathogenesis of osteoporosis: concepts, conflicts, and prospects. J Clin Invest 2005; 115: 3318–25.

16. Lee K, Jessop H, Suswillo R et al. Endocrinology: bone adaptation requires oestrogen receptor-alpha. Nature 2003; 424: 389.

17. Colston KW, King RWB, Hayward J et al. Estrogen receptors and human bone cells: immuno cytochemical studies. J Bone Miner Res 1989; 4: 625–31.

18. Windahl SH, Hollberg K, Vidal O et al. Female estrogen receptor beta–/– mice are partially protected against age-related trabecular bone loss. J Bone Miner Res 2001; 16: 1388–98.

19. Sims NA, Dupont S, Krust A et al. Deletion of estrogen receptors reveals a regulatory role for estrogen receptors-beta in bone remodeling in females but not in males. Bone 2002; 30: 18–25.

20. Gao Y, Qian WP, Dark K et al. Estrogen prevents bone loss through transforming growth factor beta signaling in T cells. Proc Natl Acad Sci USA 2004; 101: 16618–23.

21. Hughes DE, Dai A, Tiffee JC et al. Estrogen promotes apoptosis of murine osteoclasts mediated by TGF-beta. Nat Med 1996; 2: 1132–6.

22. Russell RGG, Bunning RAD, Hughes DE et al. Humoral and local factors affecting bone formation and resorption. In: Stevenson J, ed. New Techniques in Metabolic Bone Disease. London: Wright, 1990: 1–20.

23. Stevenson JC, Abeyasekera G, Hillyard CJ et al. Regulation of calcium-regulating hormones by exogenous sex steroids in early postmenopause. Eur J Clin Invest 1983; 13: 481–7.

24. Stevenson JC, Abeyasekera G, Hillyard CJ et al. Calcitonin and the calcium-regulating hormones in postmenopausal women: effect of oestrogens. Lancet 1981; 1: 693–5.

25. Delorme ML, Digioia Y, Fandard J et al. Oestrogens et calcitonie. Ann d'Endo 1976; 37: 503–4.

26. Hillyard CJ, Stevenson JC, MacIntyre I. Relative deficiency of plasma-calcitonin in normal women. Lancet 1978; 1: 961–2.

27. Tiegs RD, Barta J, Heath H. Does oral contraceptive therapy affect calcitonin secretion in premenopausal women? Presented at The Endocrine Society, 67th Annual General Meeting, Baltimore, MD, 1985; 50.

28. Taggart HM, Chesnut CH IIIrd, Ivey JL et al. Deficient calcitonin response to calcium stimulation in postmenopausal osteoporosis. Lancet 1982; 1: 475–8.

29. Tiegs RD, Body JJ, Wahner HW et al. Calcitonin secretion in postmenopausal osteoporosis. N Engl J Med 1985; 312: 1097–100.

30. Pacifici R, Rifas L, Teitelbaum S et al. Spontaneous release of interleukin-1 from human blood monocytes reflects bone formation in idiopathic bone osteoporosis. Proc Natl Acad Sci USA 1987; 84: 4616–20.

31. Ralston SH. Analysis of gene expression in human bone biopsies by polymerase chain reaction: evidence for enhanced cytokine expression in postmenopausal osteoporosis. J Bone Miner Res 1994; 8: 83–90.

32. Bertolini DR, Nedwin GE, Bringman TS et al. Stimulation of bone resorption and inhibition of bone formation in vitro by human tumor necrosis factors. Nature 1986; 319: 516–21.

33. Kimble RB, Matayoshi AB, Vannice JL et al. Simultaneous block of interleukin-1 and tumor necrosis factor is required to completely prevent bone loss in the early postovariectomy period. Endocrinology 1995; 136: 3054–61.

34. Kalu DN, Salerno E, Higami Y et al. In vivo effects of transforming growth factor-beta 2 in ovariectomized rats. Bone Miner 1993; 22: 209–20.

35. Hughes DE, Dai A, Tiffee JC et al. Estrogen promotes apoptosis of murine osteoclasts mediated by TGF-beta. Nat Med 1996; 2: 1132–6.

36. Ralston SH, Ho LP, Helfrich MH et al. Nitric oxide: a cytokine-induced regulator of bone resorption. J Bone Miner Res 1995; 10: 1040–9.

37. Ralston SH, Todd D, Helfrich MH et al. Human osteoblast-like cells produce nitric oxide and express inducible nitric oxide synthase. Endocrinology 1994; 135: 330–6.

38. Ralston SH, Grabowski PS. Mechanisms of cytokine-induced bone resorption; role of nitric oxide, cyclic guanosine monophosphate and prostaglandins. Bone 1996; 19: 29–33.

39. Evans DM, Ralston SH. Nitric oxide and bone. J Bone Miner Res 1996; 11: 300–5.

40. Schlesinger PH, Mattsson JP, Blair HC. Osteoclastic acid transport: mechanism and implications for physiological and pharmacological regulation. Miner Electrolyte Metab 1994; 20: 31–9.

41. David P, Nguyen H, Barbier A et al. The bisphosphonate tiludronate is a potent inhibitor of the osteoclast vacuolar H(+)-ATPase. J Bone Miner Res 1996; 11: 1498–507.

42. Suda T, Takahashi N, Udagawa N et al. Modulation of osteoclast differentiation and function by the new members of the tumor necrosis factor receptor and ligand families. Endocr Rev 1999; 20: 345–57.

43. Bekker PJ, Holloway DL, Rasmussen AS et al. A single-dose placebo-controlled study of AMG 162, a fully human monoclonal antibody to RANKL, in postmenopausal women. J Bone Miner Res 2004; 19: 1059–66.

44. Khosla S, Amighi HM, Melton LJ et al. Correlates of osteoprotegerin levels in women and men. Osteoporos Int 2002; 13: 394–9.

45. Khosla S, Riggs BL, Atkinson EJ et al. Relationship of estrogen receptor genotypes to bone mineral density and to rates of bone loss in men. J Clin Endocrinol Metab 2004; 89: 1808–16.

46. Syed F, Khosla S. Mechanisms of sex steroid effects on bone. Biochem Biophys Res Commun 2005; 328: 688–96.

Pathophysiology

The major factors that determine whether a person develops osteoporosis are the maximum (peak) bone density that is achieved and the amount that is subsequently lost. Bone quality and architecture are also important.

PEAK BONE MASS

Peak bone mass in men and women is probably achieved soon after their skeletal growth ceases[1,2] (Figures 3.1 and 3.2). The bone mass at skeletal maturity differs between the sexes, being 30–50% greater in men than in women[3,4]. However, the lean/bone mass ratios in mature men and women are similar, suggesting that both sexes at that time have an equal capacity to withstand mechanical trauma.

Peak bone mass is largely determined by genetic factors. The variance in bone mineral density between dizygotic twins is much greater than in monozygotic twins[5], and the daughters of women who have had a hip fracture have lower than average bone mineral density[6]. Genetic factors are almost certainly the reason for racial differences in bone mineral density, with a higher bone mineral density in blacks compared with whites[7] and no evidence of a change in the incidence of osteoporosis in people who migrate from an area of low incidence to one of high incidence.

Environmental influences on peak bone mass include diet and exercise. Some studies suggest that calcium intake during childhood and adolescence influences peak bone mass[8–10], but there is little evidence that calcium supplementation in school-age children has any effect[11]. It is possible that general dietary intake in early life is as important as calcium intake as a determinant of peak bone mass[11].

Although it is well established that long-term physical exercise results in regional increases in bone mass[12] (Figure 3.3) and immobilization leads to bone loss, it is uncertain whether a lifetime of activity reduces the risk of hip fracture[12,14]. Surprisingly few studies have examined the effect of exercise in early adult life on peak bone mass. A preliminary study by Kanders and colleagues[8] suggested that both an adequate intake of calcium and an active lifestyle are necessary for maximizing bone mineral density in early adult life. Data from a UK study suggest that, after allowing for body build, physical activity is the major determinant of peak bone density[15]. A recent study that attempted to explain variance in peak bone mineral density reported that vitamin D receptor (VDR), estrogen receptor (ER)α, and collagen type Iα1 (COLIα1) genes and other factors such as birth weight, lifestyle, diet, and exercise were not major factors, and that the important genetic and environmental influences remain to be found[16].

Excessive exercise may lead to hypothalamic-induced hypoestrogenism which, in turn, results in reduced bone mineral density[17–19]. Thus, physical activity cannot counteract the effects of hormone deprivation on the skeleton. Prolonged periods of hypoestrogenism during young adult life, such as are seen in anorexia nervosa, reduce peak bone density and predispose to osteoporosis.

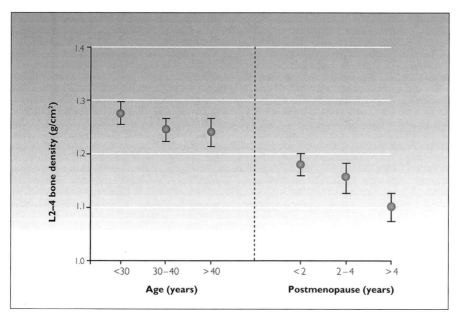

Figure 3.1 Bone density in the lumbar spine (L2–4) in 107 premenopausal and 166 postmenopausal healthy women according to age or time since menopause. There is rapid loss of bone density following the menopause. From reference 2, with permission

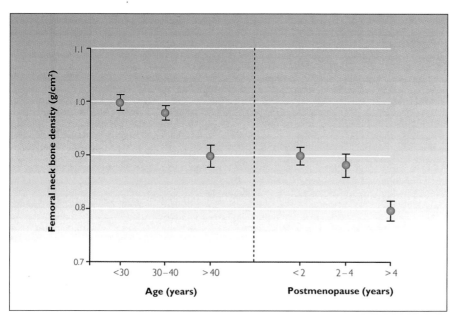

Figure 3.2 Bone density in the femoral neck in 108 premenopausal and 171 postmenopausal healthy women according to age or time since menopause. There is some premenopausal loss of bone density, but more rapid loss following the menopause. From reference 2, with permission

SMOKING, ALCOHOL, AND LIFESTYLE FACTORS

Smoking is associated with a reduced peak bone mass[2,20], earlier menopause[21], and thinness[22], all of which are risk factors for osteoporotic fracture. It appears to reduce bone mineral density by a mechanism that is independent of its effect on weight or estrogen metabolism[20], and may act by reducing calcium absorption[23,24]. Data from a twin study suggest that women who smoke 20 cigarettes a day throughout adulthood will, by the time of the menopause, have an average bone mineral density deficit of 5–10% compared with non-smokers[25].

It is not known whether the lower bone mineral density found in alcoholics[26] is mainly due to inadequate dietary intake, poor exercise, or a direct effect of alcohol in reducing osteoblastic activity[27], but it is likely to be a combination of these factors. Although the bone mineral density in the proximal femur has been shown to be significantly lower in premenopausal women who consume more than two drinks per day compared with those who consume less[2], the differences are

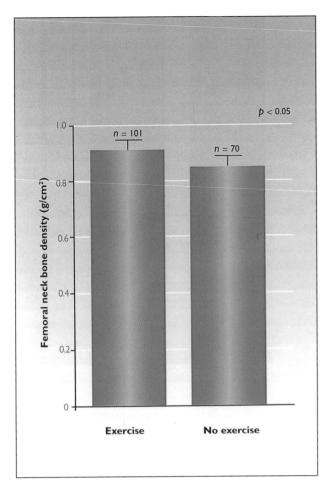

Figure 3.3 Difference in femoral neck bone density between 101 healthy postmenopausal women who took regular weight-bearing exercise and 70 who did not. From reference 13, with permission

small. A Finnish study of risk factors for fracture in 3140 women followed up for a mean of 2.4 years showed greater alcohol intake in those who developed fracture than those who did not[28]. This finding may be due to an effect of alcohol on balance rather than bone mineral density. A recent study of predictors of bone loss from the Framingham cohort demonstrated that an alcohol intake of 207 ml or more ($\geq$ 7 fl oz) per week is a risk factor for bone loss, but concluded that weight, estrogen use, and cigarette smoking were the most important predictors of bone health[29].

Increased parity is associated with increased bone mineral density. A retrospective UK study[30] of 825 women found a 1% gain in bone mineral density per live birth that was independent of other risk factors.

VITAMIN D

The active form of vitamin D, 1,25-dihydroxyvitamin D ($1,25(OH)_2D$), has important physiologic activities, including upregulating intestinal calcium and phosphate absorption. Inadequate vitamin D levels lead to impaired calcium absorption and a compensatory increase in parathyroid hormone (PTH) levels. This results in increased bone resorption and accelerated bone loss[31,32].

Vitamin D may also have a direct effect on muscle strength and dexterity. Receptors for $1,25(OH)_2D$ have been identified in skeletal muscle tissue[33–35] and low vitamin D levels have been associated with myopathy in patients with osteomalacia[36]. There appears to be a relationship between low serum vitamin D and age-related muscle weakness[37], increased body sway[38], increased risk of falls[39–42], and fall-related fractures[38].

BONE LOSS

Although one study[43] suggested that integral spinal bone mineral density declines linearly throughout life, and another[44] found that at least 50% of trabecular bone in women is lost before the menopause, most authorities agree that bone mineral density declines slowly in women until just before the menopause and that the loss increases considerably thereafter[45] (see Figures 3.1 and 3.2). Bone loss probably begins in the third or fourth decade of life and may be due, at least in men, to a decline in osteoblast function[45]. The decline in bone mineral density is around 0.5% per year.

In women, bone mineral density appears to fall exponentially, commencing just before the menopause[46,47] when ovarian function begins to decline. This loss is chiefly due to the increased resorption of bone[48–51] superimposed on the effects of aging. The loss of bone is greatest initially and may be as much as 5% per year for vertebral trabecular bone[52,53]. The loss is even greater after oophorectomy[54]. The loss of cortical bone in the perimenopausal years is slower than for trabecular bone[52,55–57], and, after 8–10 years, the rate of total bone loss declines to less than 1% per annum.

There is accumulating evidence that the rate of perimenopausal bone loss varies considerably between women. Approximately 35% of women lose large amounts of bone mineral at the menopause; they are the 'fast' bone losers. A fast rate of bone loss and a low bone mineral density may contribute equally to future risk of fracture[58]. Fast bone losers may lose approximately 50% more bone mass at the wrist, spine, and hip within 12 years of the menopause than slow bone losers[59]. Some reports suggest that this difference is not related to initial bone mineral content, parity, or smoking habits, but to estrogen levels and fat mass[60]. Fat postmenopausal women have higher endogenous estrogen production[61,62], and it appears that fast bone losers have lower serum concentrations of estrogens than slow bone losers[63–65]. Some authors have demonstrated that perimenopausal white women with the highest bone masses lose most bone, in absolute terms, following the loss of ovarian function[54,55]. However, a prospective UK follow-up study of postmenopausal women over 5 years found no correlation between rate of bone loss in the forearm and spine and baseline bone density[66].

BONE ARCHITECTURE AND QUALITY

The structural architecture of bone has received little attention until fairly recently. Recent research has focused upon trabecular bone loss and its response to treatment, as it is this bone type that shows the greatest metabolic activity (Figures 3.4–3.7). Trabecular bone loss may result from thinning or loss of trabeculae. The latter leads to a reduction in 'connectedness' of the bone elements (Figures 3.8 and 3.9), which may then have no functional value, but will contribute to the bone mineral density. However, there is evidence that a reduced connectedness is also associated with a greater reduction in bone mineral density than is trabecular thinning[67]. Both processes appear to occur with advancing age in both sexes, but disconnectedness is found more often in women[68]. Some data suggest that trabecular thinning is due to reduced bone formation,

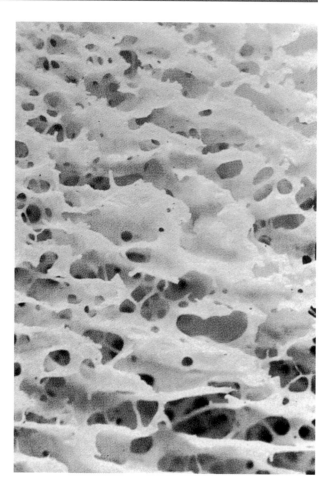

Figure 3.4 Typical isotropic trabecular (or cancellous) bone from a non-weight-bearing part of the skeleton (iliac crest). The tissue forms a three-dimensional lattice of anastomosing plates and struts without a fixed orientation in space. This structure provides the maximum support with a minimum of material. Courtesy of Dr Leif Mosekilde

whereas erosion is secondary to increased bone turnover, which occurs during the perimenopausal years[69]. Increased bone turnover by itself will increase fracture risk because of an increased likelihood of trabecular perforation. Conversely, therapeutic reductions in bone turnover may reduce fracture risk even before significant increases in density have been achieved.

Computed analysis of the structure of iliac crest bone biopsies have made possible the measurement of indices of bone architecture such as trabecular pattern, trabecular separation, and number[70]. Such techniques have been used for detailed study of the effects of the menopause and its treatment on bone architecture[71–73].

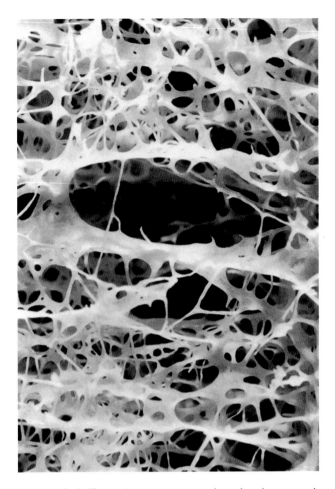

Figure 3.5 Typical anisotropic trabecular (or cancellous) bone from a weight-bearing part of the skeleton (spine). The tissue forms a three-dimensional lattice of thick anastomosing columns and thinner horizontal struts. Courtesy of Dr Leif Mosekilde

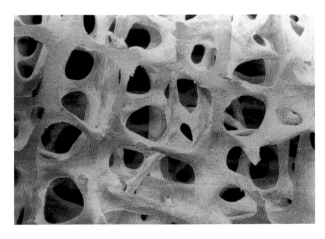

Figure 3.6 Scanning electron micrograph (SEM) of normal trabecular bone showing thick trabecular plates, which are all interconnected. Courtesy of Professor Alan Boyde

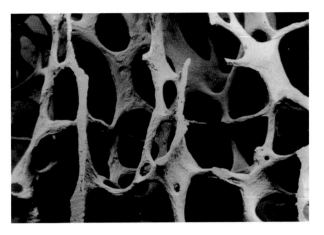

Figure 3.7 SEM of osteoporotic trabecular bone showing marked thinning and disconnection of trabeculae. Courtesy of Professor Alan Boyde

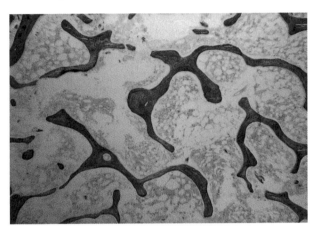

Figure 3.8 Histological biopsy section of iliac crest bone (Goldner's trichrome) from a non-osteoporotic subject shows connectivity of the trabecular elements. Courtesy of Dr David Dempster

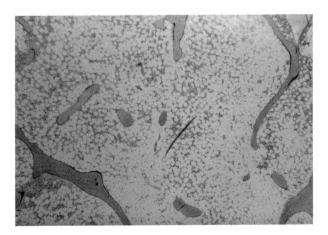

Figure 3.9 Histological biopsy section of iliac crest bone (Goldner's trichrome) from a patient with osteoporosis shows marked loss of trabecular elements. Courtesy of Dr David Dempster

REFERENCES

1. Wasnich RD, Ross PD, Davis JW, Vogel JM. A comparison of single and multisite BMC measurements for assessment of spine fracture probability. J Nucl Med 1989; 30: 1166–71.

2. Stevenson JC, Lees B, Devenport M et al. Determinants of bone density in normal women: risk factors for future osteoporosis? BMJ 1989; 298: 924–8.

3. Thomsen K, Gotfredsen A, Christiansen C. Is postmenopausal bone loss an age-related phenomenon? Calcif Tissue Int 1986; 39: 132–27.

4. Guesens P, Dequeker J, Verstraeten A et al. Age, sex- and menopause-related changes of vertebral and peripheral bone: population study using dual-photon absorptiometry and radiogrammetry. J Nucl Med 1986; 27: 1540–9.

5. Smith DM, Nance WE, Kang KW et al. Genetic factors in determining bone mass. J Clin Invest 1973; 52: 2800–8.

6. Seeman E, Tsalamandris C, Formica C et al. Reduced femoral neck bone density in the daughters of women with hip fractures: the role of low peak bone density in the pathogenesis of osteoporosis. J Bone Miner Res 1994; 9: 739–43.

7. Cohn SH, Abesamis C, Yamasura S et al. Comparative skeletal mass and radial bone mineral content in black and white women. Metabolism 1977; 26: 171–8.

8. Kanders B, Lindsay R, Dempster DW et al. Determinants of bone mass in young healthy women. In: Christiansen C, ed. Osteoporosis. Aalborg: Stiftsbogtrykkeri, 1984: 337–40.

9. Sandler RB, Slemenda CW, LaPorte RE et al. Postmenopausal bone density and milk consumption in childhood and adolescence. Am J Clin Nutr 1985; 42: 270–4.

10. Soroko S, Holbrook TL, Edelstein S et al. Lifetime milk consumption and bone mineral density in older women. Am J Public Health 1994; 84: 1319–22.

11. Kanis JA, Passmore R. Calcium supplementation of the diet-1. BMJ 1989; 298: 137–40.

12. Greendale GA, Barrett-Connor E, Edelstein S et al. Lifetime leisure exercise and osteoporosis. The Rancho Bernardo study. Am J Epidemiol 1995; 141: 951–9.

13. Stevenson JC, Less B, Fielding C et al. Exercise and the skeleton. In Smith R, ed. Osteoporosis. London: Royal College of Physicians, 1990: 119–24.

14. Jaglal SB, Kreiger N, Darlington GA. Lifetime occupational physical activity and risk of hip fracture in women. Ann Epidemiol 1995; 5: 321–4.

15. Cooper C, Cawley M, Bhalla A et al. Childhood growth, physical activity, and peak bone mass in women. J Bone Miner Res 1995; 10: 940–7.

16. McGuigan FEA, Murray L, Gallagher A et al. Genetic and environmental determinants of peak bone mass in young men and women. J Bone Miner Res 2002; 17: 1273–9.

17. Lloyd T, Myers C, Buchanan JR, Demers LM. Collegiate women athletes with irregular menses during adolescence have decreased bone density. Obstet Gynecol 1988; 72: 639–42.

18. Lindberg JS, Fears WB, Hunt MM et al. Exercise induced amenorrhea and bone density. Ann Intern Med 1984; 101: 258–60.

19. Drinkwater BL, Nilson K, Chesnut CH IIIrd et al. Bone mineral density of amenorrheic and eumenorrheic athletes. N Engl J Med 1984; 311: 277–81.

20. Slemender CW, Hui SL, Longcope C, Johnson CC. Cigarette smoking. Obesity and bone mass. J Bone Miner Res 1989; 4: 737–41.

21. Baron BA. Smoking and estrogen-related disease. Am J Epidemiol 1984; 119: 9–22.

22. Rigotti NA. Cigarette smoking and body weight. N Engl J Med 1989; 320: 931–3.

23. Krall EA, Dawson-Hughes B. Smoking increases bone loss and decreases intestinal calcium absorption. J Bone Miner Res 1999; 14: 215–20.

24. Law MR, Hackshaw AK. A meta-analysis of cigarette smoking, bone mineral density and risk of hip fracture: recognition of a major effect. BMJ 1997; 315: 841–6.

25. Hopper JL, Seeman E. The bone density of female twins discordant for tobacco use. N Engl J Med 1994; 330: 387–92.

26. Saville PD. Changes in bone mass with age and alcoholism. J Bone Joint Surg 1965; 47: 492–9.

27. De Vernejoul MC, Bielakoff J, Herve M et al. Evidence for defective osteoblastic function. A role for alcohol and tobacco consumption in osteoporosis in middle aged men. Clin Orthop 1983; 179: 107–15.

28. Tuppurainen M, Kroger H, Honkanen R et al. Risks of perimenopausal fractures – a prospective population-based study. Acta Obstet Gynecol Scand 1995; 74: 624–8.

29. Hannan MT, Felson DT, Dawson-Hughes B et al. Risk factors for longitudinal bone loss in elderly men and women: the Framingham Osteoporosis Study. J Bone Miner Res 2000; 15: 710–20.

30. Murphy S, Shaw KT, May H, Compston JE. Parity and bone density in middle age women. Osteoporos Int 1994; 4: 162–6.

31. Prince RL, Dick I, Devine A et al. The effects of menopause and age on calcitropic hormones: a cross-sectional study of 655 healthy women aged 35 to 90. J Bone Miner Res 1995; 10: 835–42.

32. Brazier M, Kamel S, Maamer M et al. The markers of bone remodeling in the elderly subject: effects of vitamin D insufficiency and its correction. J Bone Miner Res 1995; 10: 1753–61.

33. Simpson RU, Thomas GA, Arnold AJ. Identification of 1,25-dihydroxyvitamin D3 receptors and activities in muscle. J Biol Chem 1985; 260: 8882–91.

34. Costa EM, Blau HM, Feldman D. 1,25-dihydroxyvitamin D3 receptors and hormonal responses in cloned human skeletal muscle cells. Endocrinology 1986; 119: 2214–20.

35. Haddad JG, Walgate J, Min C, Hahn TJ. Vitamin D metabolite binding proteins in human tissue. Biochem Biophys Acta 1976; 444: 921–5.

36. Schott G, Wills M. Muscle weakness in osteomalacia. Lancet 1976; 2: 626–9.

37. Boland R. Role of vitamin D in skeletal muscle function. Endocr Rev 1986; 7: 434–8.

38. Pfeifer M, Begerow B, Minne HW et al. Vitamin D status, trunk muscle strength, body sway, falls, and fractures among 237 postmenopausal women with osteoporosis. Exp Clin Endocrinol Diabetes 2001; 109: 87–92.

39. Sambrook PN, Chen JS, March LM et al. Serum parathyroid hormone predicts time to fall independent of vitamin D status in a frail elderly population. J Clin Endocrinol Metab 2004; 89: 1572–6.

40. Bischoff-Ferrari HA, Dawson-Hughes B, Willett WC et al. Effect of vitamin D on falls: a meta-analysis. JAMA 2004; 291: 1999–2006.

41. Bischoff HA, Stahelin HB, Dick W et al. Effects of vitamin D and calcium supplementation on falls: a randomized controlled trial. J Bone Miner Res 2003; 18: 343–51.

42. Dukas L, Bischoff HA, Lindpainter LS et al. Alfacalcidol reduces the number of fallers in a community-dwelling elderly population with a minimum calcium intake of more than 500 mg daily. J Am Geriatr Soc 2004; 52: 230–6.

43. Riggs BL, Wahner HW, Seeman E et al. Changes in bone mineral density of the proximal femur and spine with aging. Differences between the post-menopausal and senile osteoporosis syndromes. J Clin Invest 1982; 70: 716–23.

44. Riggs BL, Wahner HW, Dunn WL et al. Differential changes in bone mineral density of the appendicular and axial skeleton with aging: relationship to spinal osteoporosis. J Clin Invest 1981; 67: 328–35.

45. Nordin BEC, Marshall DH, Francis RM, Crilly RG. The effect of sex steroid and corticosteroid hormones on bone. J Steroid Biochem 1981; 15: 171–4.

46. Abdallah H, Hart DM, Lindsay R. Differential bone loss and effects of long-term oestrogen therapy according to time of introduction of therapy after oophorectomy. In: Christiansen C, Arnaud C, Nordin B et al, eds. Osteoporosis. Glostrup: Glostrup Hospital, 1984: 621–3.

47. Krolner B, Nielsen SP. Bone mineral content of the lumbar spine in normal and osteoporotic women: cross-sectional and longitudinal studies. Clin Sci 1982; 62: 329–36.

48. Riggs BL, Jowsey J, Kelly PJ et al. Effect of sex hormones on bone in primary osteoporosis. J Clin Invest 1969; 48: 1065–72.

49. Nordin BEC, Aaron J, Speed R, Crilly RG. Bone formation and resorption as the determinants of trabecular bone volume in postmenopausal osteoporosis. Lancet 1981; 2: 277–9.

50. Heaney RP, Recker RR, Saville PD. Menopausal changes in bone remodelling. J Lab Clin Med 1978; 92: 964–70.

51. Hansen JW, Gordan GS, Prussin SG. Direct measurement of osteolysis in man. J Clin Invest 1973; 52: 304–15.

52. Stevenson JC, Banks LM, Spinks TJ et al. Regional and total skeletal measurements in the early postmenopause. J Clin Invest 1987; 80: 258–62.

53. Ettinger B, Genant HK, Cann CE. Postmenopausal bone loss is prevented by treatment with low

dosage estrogen with calcium. Ann Intern Med 1987; 106: 40–5.

54. Stevenson JC, Lees B, Banks LM, Whitehead MI. Assessment of therapeutic options for prevention of bone loss. In: Christiansen C, Johansen J, Riis BJ, eds. Osteoporosis. Viborg: Norhaven Bogtrykken A/S, 1987: 392–3.

55. Genant HK, Cann CE, Ettinger B, Gordan GS. Quantitative computed tomography of vertebral spongiosa: a sensitive method of detecting early bone loss after oophorectomy. Ann Intern Med 1982; 97: 699–705.

56. Christiansen C, Christiansen MS, Transbøl I. Bone mass in postmenopausal women after withdrawal of oestrogen replacement therapy. Lancet 1981; 1: 459–61.

57. Lindsay R, Hart DM, Aitken JM et al. Long-term prevention of postmenopausal osteoporosis by oestrogen. Lancet 1976; 1: 1038–41.

58. Riis BJ. The role of bone loss. Am J Med 1995; 98: 29S–32S.

59. Christiansen C. What should be done at the time of menopause? Am J Med 1995; 98: 56S–9S.

60. Christiansen C, Riis BJ, Rødbro P. Prediction of rapid bone loss in postmenopausal women. Lancet 1987; 1: 1105–7.

61. Poortman J, Thijssen JHH, de Waard F. Plasma oestrone, oestradiol and androstanedione levels in postmenopausal women: relation to body weight and height. Maturitas 1981; 3: 65–71.

62. MacDonald PC, Edman CD, Hemsell DL et al. Effect of obesity on conversion of plasma androstanedione to estrone in postmenopausal women with and without endometrial cancer. Am J Obstet Gynecol 1978; 130: 448–55.

63. Christiansen C. Prophylactic treatment for age-related bone loss in women. In: Christiansen C, Arnaud CD, Nordin BEC et al, eds. Proceedings of the International Symposium on Osteoporosis. Copenhagen: Aalborg Stiftsbogtrykkeri, 1984; 2: 587–93.

64. Johnston CC Jr, Hui SL, Witt RM et al. Early menopausal changes in bone mass and sex steroids. J Clin Endocrinol Metab 1985; 61: 905–11.

65. Slemender C, Hui SL, Longcope C, Johnston CC. Sex steroids and bone mass: a study about the time of menopause. J Clin Invest 1987; 80: 1261–9.

66. Clements D, Compston JE, Evans C, Evans WD. Bone loss in normal British women; a 5-year follow-up. Br J Radiol 1993; 66: 1134–7.

67. Pugh JW, Rose RM, Radin EL. Elastic and viscoelastic properties of bone. J Biomech 1973; 6: 475–85.

68. Compston JE, Mellish RWE, Garrahan NJ. Age-related changes in the iliac crest trabecular micro-anatomic bone structure in man. Bone 1978; 8: 289–92.

69. Compston JE. Structural mechanisms of trabecular bone loss. In: Smith R, ed. Osteoporosis. London: Royal College of Physicians, 1990: 35–43.

70. Chappard D, Legrand E, Haettich B et al. Fractal dimension of trabecular bone: comparison of three histomorphometric computed techniques for measuring the architectural two-dimensional complexity. J Pathol 2001; 195: 515–21.

71. Oka K, Kumasaka S, Kashima I. Assessment of bone feature parameters from lumbar trabecular skeletal patterns using mathematical morphology image processing. J Bone Miner Metab 2002; 20: 201–8.

72. Banse X, Devogelaer JP, Lafosse A et al. Cross-link profile of bone collagen correlates with structural organization of trabeculae. Bone 2002; 31: 70–6.

73. Miki T, Nakatsuka K, Naka H et al. Effect and safety of intermittent weekly administration of human parathyroid hormone 1-34 in patients with primary osteoporosis evaluated by histomorphometry and microstructural analysis of iliac trabecular bone before and after 1 year of treatment. J Bone Miner Metab 2004; 22: 569–76.

CHAPTER 4

Biochemical changes

CALCIUM, VITAMIN D, AND PARATHYROID HORMONE

In the normal person whose bone mass is being maintained, approximately 6 mmol of calcium enters and leaves the skeleton each day[1], and the amount of calcium leaving the body in the urine and digestive juices is matched by the amount absorbed from the gut. Plasma calcium is chiefly regulated by the actions of parathyroid hormone, and vitamin D and its derivatives, on the kidney, skeleton, and gut.

Parathyroid hormone secretion increases in response to a fall in plasma calcium and acts directly on the kidney to increase tubular calcium reabsorption. It increases renal synthesis of 1,25-dihydroxyvitamin D which then acts on the gut to increase the active transport of calcium. Increasing parathyroid hormone levels result in increased bone turnover, with resorption predominating when parathyroid hormone levels become supraphysiological. An increase in serum calcium reduces parathyroid hormone secretion and stimulates the release of calcitonin.

Calcium metabolism changes considerably around the time of the menopause. Both bone resorption and bone formation increase, but with formation less so than resorption, leading to a negative calcium balance of approximately 50 mg/day. This calcium is excreted in the urine. The plasma calcium rises at the menopause[2], leading to a small homeostatic decline in levels of both parathyroid hormone and 1,25-dihydroxyvitamin D in early postmenopausal women[3]. The lower level of 1,25-dihydroxyvitamin D, in turn, results in a fall in intestinal calcium absorption[4]. Compared with normal subjects, osteoporotic women show differences in calcium balance, plasma calcium, and calcium-regulating hormones similar to those between pre- and postmenopausal women[4,5]. This suggests that neither a primary defect in calcium absorption[6] nor renal endocrine failure[7] is the cause of osteoporosis in the majority of cases.

Urinary calcium excretion

The early morning urinary fasting calcium-to-creatinine ratio may reflect the difference between bone resorption and formation, as the influence of intestinal calcium absorption is minimal. Fasting urinary calcium-to-creatinine ratios increase after the menopause and fall in response to antiresorption therapy.

BIOCHEMICAL MARKERS OF BONE FORMATION

Alkaline phosphatase

The principal role of alkaline phosphatase is probably to hydrolyze pyrophosphate, and therefore permit growth of hydroxyapatite crystals on newly synthesized mineralizing osteoid[8]. Levels of serum alkaline phosphatase are raised by increased bone turnover due to increased osteoblastic production[9] (Figure 4.1) but, as there are many

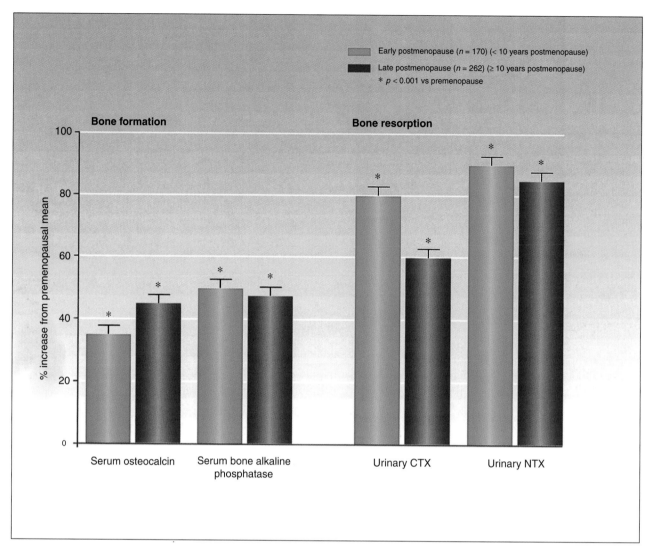

Figure 4.1 Levels of bone formation and bone resorption markers are increased in both early (within 10 years of the menopause; mean 5 years) and late (10 years or more postmenopause; mean 20 years; range 10–40 years) postmenopausal women (n = 432). For each marker in each group, mean levels are expressed as a percentage increase (± SEM) over the mean of 134 premenopausal women (ages 31–57 years). Both bone formation and resorption were markedly increased at the time of menopause, and a high bone turnover is maintained in late post-menopausal women and in the elderly. NTX, type I cross-linked N telopeptides; CTX, type I C telopeptide break-down products. Adapted from reference 9, with permission

non-bony causes of elevated serum alkaline phosphatase levels, interpretation is difficult. Assays of bone-specific alkaline phosphatase have been developed using chemical inhibition[10], gel electrophoresis[11], and heat inactivation[12]. The generation of specific monoclonal antibodies to bone isoenzymes should lead to even more sensitive tests in the future[13,14].

Procollagen extension peptides

During the formation of collagen from procollagen, N- and C-terminal peptides are released. A molecule incorporating three C-terminal fragments (PColl-1-C) may be measured in plasma, and appears to be raised in Paget's disease, and reduced in this disease with successful treatment using calcitonin or bisphosphonate[15]. In a study of 12 osteoporotic patients[16], circulating levels of these fragments were lowered by estrogen and progestogen hormone replacement therapy (HRT). More recently, these fragments have been used extensively as markers of bone formation in studies of osteoporosis and its treatment[17–20].

Gla protein

Bone Gla protein (osteocalcin) is a non-collagenous protein synthesized exclusively by osteoblasts. It is a sensitive and specific marker of osteoblastic activity in a variety of metabolic bone diseases, including osteoporosis[21–25].

BIOCHEMICAL MARKERS OF BONE RESORPTION

Urinary hydroxyproline

Hydroxyproline is a product of collagen breakdown, and approximately 10% of the total production is excreted into the urine as the peptide-bound form. Collection of urine for the measurement of total 24-h urinary hydroxyproline is inconvenient for patients, and has to a large extent been replaced by the fasting urinary hydroxyproline-to-creatinine ratio, which may be determined from a small urine sample. Urinary hydroxyproline may be increased by meat and fish in the diet, acute infections, and collagen turnover in other tissues such as skin and cartilage, and results should be viewed with caution[8]. Urinary hydroxyproline has been largely superseded by other more specific markers of resorption[26].

Pyridinoline cross-links

Lysyl pyridinoline cross-links appear to be specific to mature type I bone collagen, and are measurable in urine because of their natural fluorescence. Urinary pyridinoline and deoxypyridinoline concentrations are directly related to bone-matrix degradation. These markers are found to be elevated in postmenopausal normal and osteoporotic women compared with premenopausal women, and reduced with estrogen replacement therapy[27–29]. Urinary pyridinoline cross-link excretion has been

reported to be superior to urinary hydroxyproline in discriminating between women with or without osteoporosis[30]. Serum levels of these markers also appear to reflect bone formation and resorption rates[31].

Type I collagen telopeptides

Carboxy-terminal telopeptides of type I collagen may be measured in serum, and appear to discriminate between osteoporotic and non-osteoporotic women[32,33]. Initial studies suggested they may not be sufficiently sensitive as markers of resorption to detect the changes induced by HRT[34], but more recent reports indicate that they are useful[35,36].

Other markers

Peripheral serum levels of IL-1 and IL-6 have, so far, not been found to be useful markers of osteoporosis[37]. Serial measurements of serum OPG after estrogen replacement therapy (ERT) appear not to be a useful predictor of the long-term effects of estrogen on bone density[35].

Biochemical markers of bone formation and resorption can be useful in indicating the state of bone turnover (Figure 4.1). However, attempts to combine markers of bone turnover to improve the sensitivity and specificity of detection of low bone mineral density have proved disappointing[38]. Although single markers may prove to be useful in monitoring treatment, the lack of accepted normal ranges and guidelines for their use make them still of limited value in the clinical setting[39].

REFERENCES

1. Peacock M. Hypercalcaemia and calcium homeostasis. Metab Bone Dis Rel Res 1980; 2: 143–50.

2. Marshall RW, Francis RM, Hodgkinson A. Plasma total and ionised calcium, albumin and globulin concentrations in pre- and postmenopausal women and the effects of oestrogen administration. Clin Chim Acta 1982; 122: 283–7.

3. Stevenson JC. Vitamin D in postmenopausal women. In: Duursma S, van der Sluys Veer J, eds. Vitamin D. Utrecht: Wetenschappelijke uitgerij Bunge, 1983: 43–55.

4. Heaney RP, Recker RR, Saville PD. Menopausal changes in calcium balance performance. J Lab Clin Med 1978; 92: 953–63.

5. Riggs BL, Jowsey J, Kelley PJ, Arnaud CD. Role of hormonal factors in the pathogenesis of post-menopausal osteoporosis. Isr J Med Sci 1976; 12: 615–19.

6. Nordin BEC. Osteomalacia, osteoporosis and calcium deficiency. Clin Orthop 1960; 17: 235–57.

7. Riggs BL, Melton LJ. Evidence for two distinct syndromes of involutional osteoporosis. Am J Med 1983; 75: 899–901.

8. Reeve J. The use of biochemical and isotopic studies in the investigation of bone disorders. In: Stevenson J, ed. New Techniques in Metabolic Bone Disease. London: Wright, 1990: 92–109.

9. Garnero P, Sornay-Rendu E, Chapuy MC, Delmas PD. Incsreased bone turnover in late postmenopausal women is a major determinant of osteoporosis. J Bone Miner Res 1996; 11: 337–49.

10. Stepan JJ, Volek V, Kolar JA. A modified inactivation inhibition method for determining the serum activity of alkaline phosphatase isoenzymes. Clin Chim Acta 1976; 69: 1–9.

11. Moss DW, King EJ. Properties of alkaline phosphatase fractions separated by starch gel electrophoresis. Biochemistry 1962; 84: 192–5.

12. Posen S, Neale FC, Clubb JS. Heat inactivation in the study of human alkaline phosphatases. Ann Intern Med 1965; 62: 1234–43.

13. Christiansen C, Riis BJ. Risk assessment using biochemical analysis. In: Smith R, ed. Osteoporosis. London: Royal College of Physicians, 1990: 158–61.

14. Eftekharian MM, Moazzeni SM, Pourfathollah AA, Khabiri, AR. Production of monoclonal antibody against alkaline phosphatase. Hum Antibodies 2005; 14: 17–21.

15. Garnero P, Delmas PD. New developments in biochemical markers for osteoporosis. Calcif Tissue Int 1996; 59(7): 2–9.

16. Hasling C, Eriksen EF, Melkko J et al. Effects of a combined estrogen–gestagen regimen on serum levels of the carboxy-terminal propeptide of human type I procollagen in osteoporosis. J Bone Miner Res 1991; 6: 1295–300.

17. Deal C, Omizo M, Schwartz EN et al. Combination teriparatide and raloxifene therapy for postmeno-pausal osteoporosis: results from a 6-month double-blind placebo-controlled trial. J Bone Miner Res 2005; 20: 1905–11.

18. Chen JS, Cameron ID, Cumming RG et al. Effect of age-related chronic immobility on markers of bone turnover. J Bone Miner Res 2006; 21: 324–31.

19. Floter A, Nathorst-Boos J, Carlstrom K et al. Effects of combined estrogen/testosterone therapy on bone and body composition in oophorectomized women. Gynecol Endocrinol 2005; 20: 155–60.

20. Dobnig H, Sipos A, Jiang Y et al. Early changes in biochemical markers of bone formation correlate with improvements in bone structure during teriparatide therapy. J Clin Endocrinol Metab 2005; 90: 3970–7.

21. Brown JP, Delmas PD, Malval L et al. Serum bone Gla protein: a specific marker for bone formation in postmenopausal osteoporosis. Lancet 1984; 1: 1091–3.

22. Miura H, Yamamoto I, Yuu I et al. Estimation of bone mineral density and bone loss by means of bone metabolic markers in postmenopausal women. Endocrinol Jpn 1995; 42: 797–802.

23. Dresner-Pollak R, Parker RA, Poku M et al. Biochemical markers of bone turnover reflect femoral bone loss in elderly women. Calcif Tissue Int 1996; 59: 328–33.

24. Greenspan SL, Resnick NM, Parker RA. Early changes in biochemical markers of bone turnover are associated with long-term changes in bone mineral density in elderly women on alendronate, hormone replacement therapy, or combination therapy: a three-year, double-blind, placebo-controlled, randomized clinical trial. J Clin Endocrinol Metab 2005; 90: 2762–7.

25. Kemmler W, Lauber D, Weineck J et al. Benefits of 2 years of intense exercise on bone density, physical fitness, and blood lipids in early post-menopausal osteopenic women: results of the Erlangen Fitness Osteoporosis Prevention Study (EFOPS). Arch Intern Med 2004; 164: 1084–91.

26. Pagani F, Francucci CM, Moro L. Markers of bone turnover: biochemical and clinical perspectives. J Endocrinol Invest 2005; 28 (10 Suppl): 8–13.

27. Seibel MJ, Cosman F, Shen V et al. Urinary hydroxy-pyridinium crosslinks of collagen as markers of bone resorption and estrogen efficacy in postmenopausal osteoporosis. J Bone Miner Res 1993; 8: 881–9.

28. Schlemmer A, Hassager C, Delmas PD et al. Urinary excretion of pyridinium cross-links in healthy women; the long-term effects of menopause and oestrogen/progesterone therapy. Clin Endocrinol 1994; 40: 777–82.

29. Okabe R, Inaba M, Nakatsuka K et al. Significance of serum CrossLaps as a predictor of changes in bone mineral density during estrogen replacement therapy; comparison with serum carboxy-terminal telopeptide of type I collagen and urinary deoxypyridinoline. J Bone Miner Metab 2004; 22: 127–31.

30. Eastell R, Robins SP, Colwel T et al. Evaluation of bone turnover in type I osteoporosis using biochemical markers specific for both bone formation and bone resorption. Osteoporos Int 1993; 3: 255–60.

31. Charles P, Mosekilde L, Risteli L et al. Assessment of bone remodelling using biochemical indicators of type I collagen synthesis and degradation: relation to calcium kinetics. Bone Miner 1994; 24: 81–94.

32. Valimaki MJ, Tahtela R, Jones JD et al. Bone resorption in healthy and osteoporotic post-menopausal women: comparison markers for serum carboxy-terminal telopeptide of type I collagen and urinary pyridinium cross-links. Eur J Endocrinol 1994; 131: 258–62.

33. Eriksen EF, Charles P, Melsen F et al. Serum markers of type I collagen formation and degradation in metabolic bone disease: correlation with bone histomorphometry. J Bone Miner Res 1993; 8: 127–32.

34. Hassager C, Jensen LT, Podenphant J et al. The carboxy-terminal pyridinoline cross-linked telopeptide of type I collagen in serum as a marker of bone resorption: the effect of nandrolone decanoate and hormone replacement therapy. Calcif Tissue Int 1994; 54: 30–3.

35. Han KO, Choi JT, Choi HA et al. The changes in circulating osteoprotegerin after hormone therapy in postmenopausal women and their relationship with oestrogen responsiveness on bone. Clin Endocrinol 2005; 62: 349–53.

36. Ravn P, Warming L, Christgau S et al. The effect on cartilage of different forms of application of postmenopausal estrogen therapy: comparison of oral and transdermal therapy. Bone 2004; 35: 1216–21.

37. Khosla S, Peterson JM, Egan K et al. Circulating cytokine levels in osteoporotic and normal women. J Clin Endocrinol Metab 1994; 79: 707–11.

38. Bettica P, Taylor AK, Talbot J et al. Clinical performances of galactosyl hydroxylysine, pyridinoline, and deoxypyridinoline in postmenopausal osteoporosis. J Clin Endocrinol Metab 1996; 81: 542–6.

39. Bonnick SL, Shulman L. Monitoring osteoporosis therapy: bone mineral density, bone turnover markers, or both? J Med 2006; 119 (4 Suppl 1): S25–31.

Diagnosis

In the past osteoporosis was often diagnosed on the basis of a low trauma fracture, for example a fall from standing, and X-ray changes. More recently, because the inverse relationship between bone mineral density (BMD) and fracture risk is now well established, the diagnosis is usually made using BMD measurements.

The World Health Organization (WHO) defines osteoporosis as a BMD 2.5 standard deviations or more below the mean value for young adults (a T score < −2.5), and severe osteoporosis as a BMD below this cut-off and one or more fragility fractures[1]. The WHO defines osteopenia as a BMD T score between −1.0 and −2.5. It should be remembered that whilst osteoporotic fracture incidence is highest in those with the most pronounced osteoporosis, a substantial number of fractures occur in women who do not have very low bone density[2,3]. A new algorithm from the WHO for the definition of osteoporosis treatment thresholds, which includes other factors such as age, is currently awaited.

RADIOGRAPHY

Radiography reveals recognizable bone loss only when 25–30% of bone density has been lost, at which time osteoporosis is generally considered to have developed. In the past, radiogrammetry has been used to assess bone mineral density of the peripheral skeleton, usually at the metacarpals. The metacarpal cortical thickness was used for many years to diagnose and predict the risk of osteoporosis. However, the sensitivity of radiography is poor[4,5], and the results of metacarpal measurement do not reflect bone mineral density at more important sites such as the hip and spine[6,7]. Although there is a correlation between bone mineral density in the peripheral and central skeleton[6] (see Figure 1.4), the association is not strong enough to predict central bone mineral density from peripheral measurements in a given subject[6,8]. At present, the main role of radiography is in the diagnosis of fractures secondary to osteoporosis (Figures 5.1–5.6).

SINGLE-PHOTON AND SINGLE X-RAY ABSORPTIOMETRY

Single-photon absorptiometry (SPA) involves passing a collimated beam of monoenergetic photons from a radioiodine (^{125}I) source through a limb and measuring the transmitted radiation, using a sodium iodide scintillation detector. There is differential absorption of photons by bone and soft tissues, which allows the total bone mineral content in the path of the beam to be calculated and expressed in grams per centimeter. The method cannot differentiate between cortical and trabecular bone, and interference from surrounding tissue limits its use to the measurement of peripheral sites, such as the distal or mid-radius. At the mid-radius, the cortical-to-trabecular bone ratio is approximately 95:5, whereas at the distal radius it is about 75:25[9]. SPA became superseded by single X-ray absorptiometry (SXA)[10]. This in turn has been superseded by dual-energy X-ray absorptiometry.

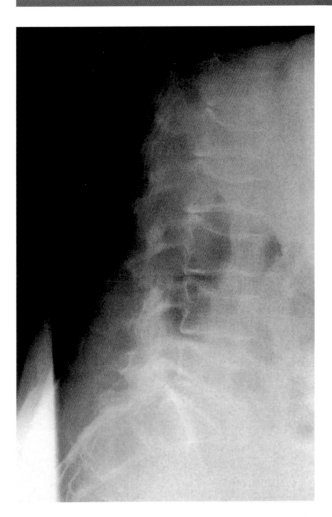

Figure 5.1 Lateral radiograph of the lumbar spine of a patient with osteoporosis shows wedging and compression of several vertebrae. Courtesy of Ms Linda Banks

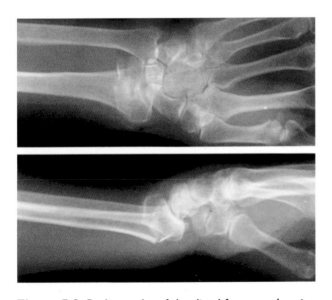

Figure 5.2 Radiographs of the distal forearm showing a Colles' fracture. Courtesy of Mr Paul Allen

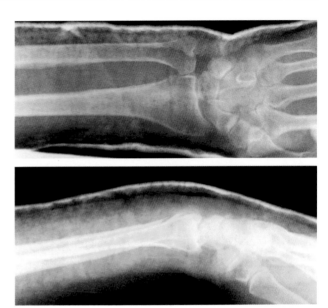

Figure 5.3 Radiographs of the distal forearm showing a Colles' fracture after reduction and external fixation. Courtesy of Mr Paul Allen

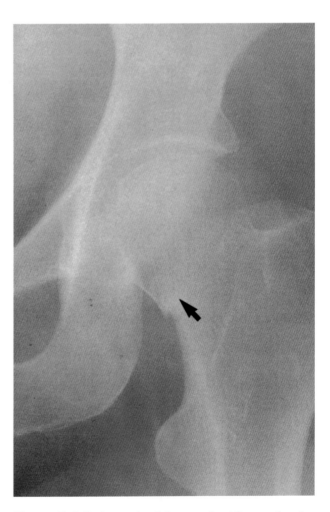

Figure 5.4 Radiograph of the proximal femur showing an intracapsular hip fracture. Courtesy of Mr Paul Allen

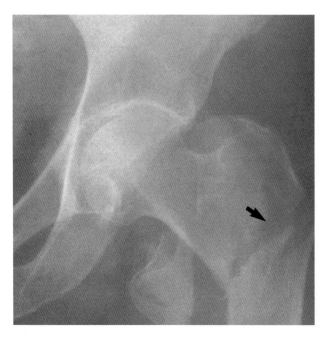

Figure 5.5 Radiograph of the proximal femur showing an extracapsular hip fracture. Courtesy of Mr Paul Allen

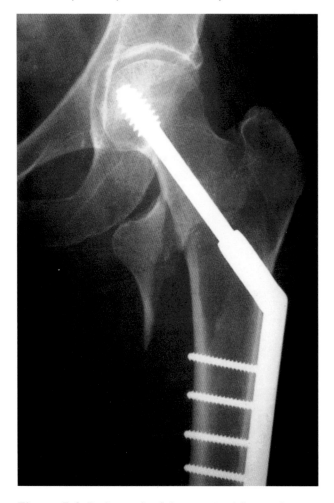

Figure 5.6 Radiograph of the proximal femur showing an extracapsular hip fracture after reduction and internal fixation. Courtesy of Mr Paul Allen

DUAL-ENERGY X-RAY ABSORPTIOMETRY

Dual-energy X-ray absorptiometry (DEXA; Figure 5.7) measures bone mineral density by determining the absorption of two beams of photons at two different energies. DEXA is able to measure bone mineral density (as mass/area) in the proximal femur and lumbar spine as well as the total body, but it cannot differentiate between cortical and trabecular bone. The cortical-to-trabecular ratio is 1:2 in the spine[11] and 3:1 in the femoral neck[12]. Thus, measurements of the total BMD at these sites are more a reflection of trabecular bone density than are measurements taken in the peripheral skeleton.

DEXA enables bone mineral density to be measured at the hip or spine with greater precision than with the methods described above (precision error: 0.5–2%). The technique is able to measure bone mineral density in the spine (Figures 5.8–5.11), proximal femur (Figures 5.12 and 5.13) and the total body (Figures 5.14 and 5.15). The scanning time is around 5 min at each site. The radiation dose is low, approximately 1 mrem for each site. Most techniques involve measurements taken from anteroposterior view. Early reports suggested that lateral views may be better than anteroposterior views in the diagnosis of osteoporosis[13], and that volumetric bone mineral density measured by DEXA from both anteroposterior and lateral views may better predict fracture than DEXA from anteroposterior view alone[14]. The precision of lateral measurement appears satisfactory[15], but these techniques have not been adopted and cannot be recommended for clinical use[16]. However, lateral views can now be used to give morphometric evaluations of vertebrae to determine vertebral deformities and fractures (Figure 5.16).

QUANTITATIVE COMPUTED TOMOGRAPHY

Quantitative computed tomography (CT; Figure 5.17) with a suitable software package enables the absorption by different calcified tissues to be determined so that areas of particular interest,

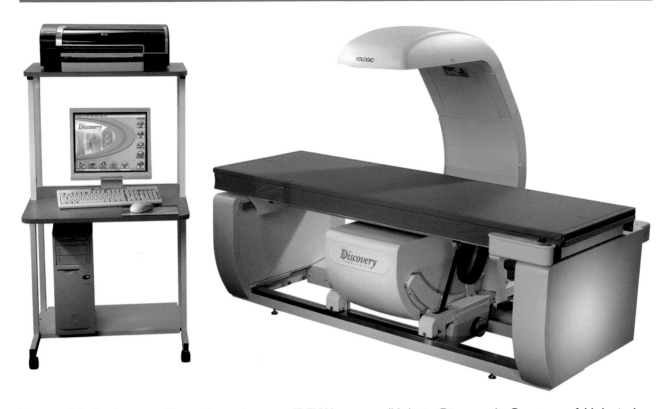

Figure 5.7 Dual-energy X-ray absorptiometry (DEXA) system (Hologic Discovery). Courtesy of Hologic Inc, Bedford, MA

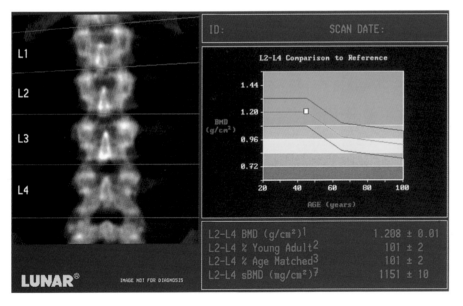

Figure 5.8 DEXA (Lunar DPX-IQ) measurements of lumbar spine bone density in a normal woman (anteroposterior (AP) view). Courtesy of GE Lunar, Madison, WI

such as the vertebral body (which has a cortical-to-trabecular ratio of approximately 5:95), may be studied[11]. The technique measures true density[11,17] with the results expressed in g/cm^3. Software automation allows accurate determination of the region of interest, and the tissue density is compared with a solid calibration phantom (Figure 5.18).

At present, CT scanning is chiefly used to assess trabecular bone density in the spine (Figure 5.19), although it has been reported to be useful in measuring radial density[18–20]. The precision and accuracy of spinal measurements are approximately 2–4% and 5–10%, respectively, but there is considerable variation depending on the method used.

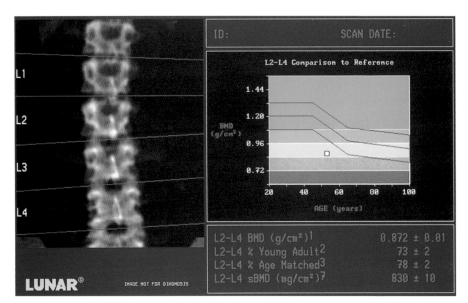

Figure 5.9 DEXA (Lunar DPX-IQ) measurements of lumbar spine bone density in an osteoporotic woman (AP view). Courtesy of GE Lunar, Madison, WI

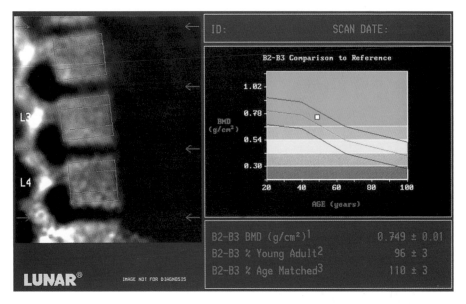

Figure 5.10 DEXA (Lunar DPX-IQ) measurements of lumbar spine bone density in a normal woman (lateral view). Courtesy of GE Lunar, Madison, WI

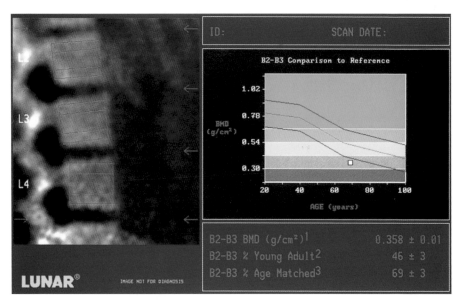

Figure 5.11 DEXA (Lunar DPX-IQ) measurements of lumbar spine bone density in an osteoporotic woman (lateral view). Courtesy of GE Lunar, Madison, WI

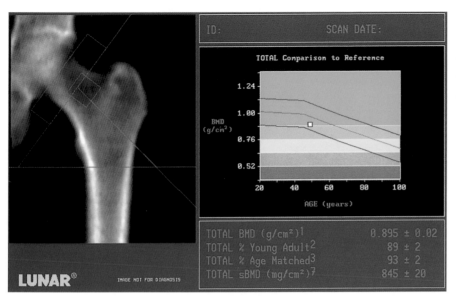

Figure 5.12 DEXA (Lunar DPX-IQ) measurements of femoral neck bone density in a normal woman (AP view). Courtesy of GE Lunar, Madison, WI

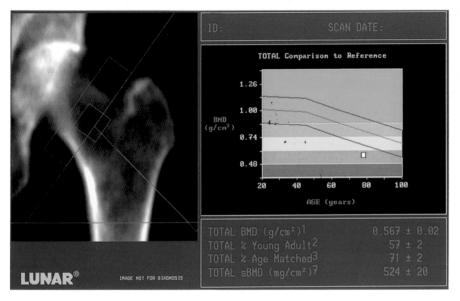

Figure 5.13 DEXA (Lunar DPX-IQ) measurements of femoral neck bone density in an osteoporotic woman (AP view). Courtesy of GE Lunar, Madison, WI

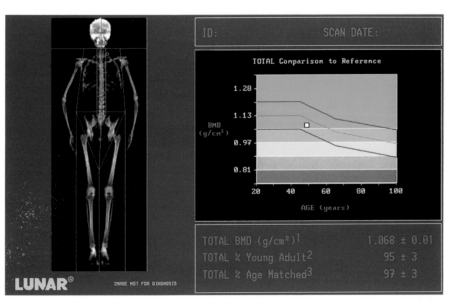

Figure 5.14 DEXA (Lunar DPX-IQ) measurements of total body bone mineral density in a normal woman (AP view). Courtesy of GE Lunar, Madison, WI

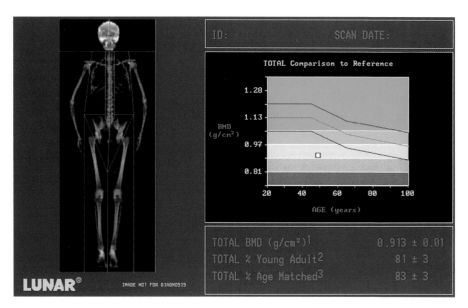

Figure 5.15 DEXA (Lunar DPX-IQ) measurements of total body bone mineral density in an osteoporotic woman (AP view). Courtesy of GE Lunar, Madison, WI

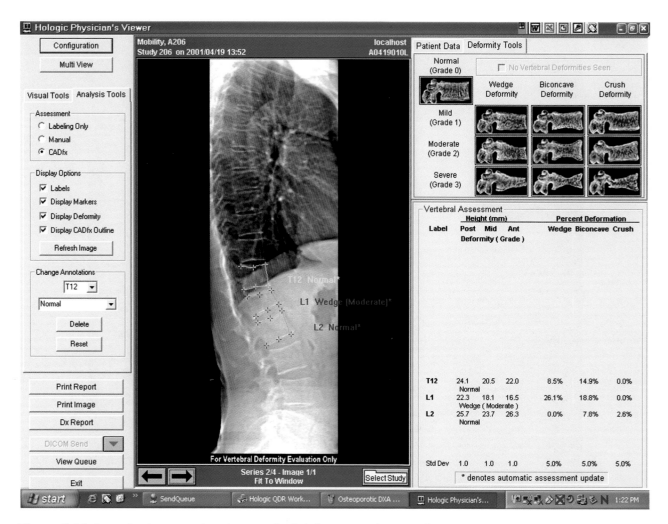

Figure 5.16 Lateral spine scan showing vertebral deformity evaluation. Courtesy of Hologic Inc, Bedford, MA

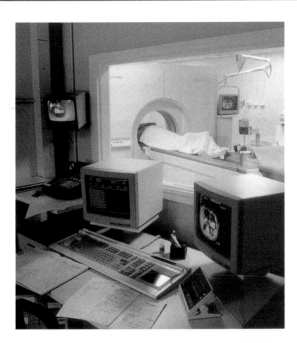

Figure 5.17 Computed tomography (CT) scanner (Siemens Somatom Plus). Courtesy of Ms Linda Banks

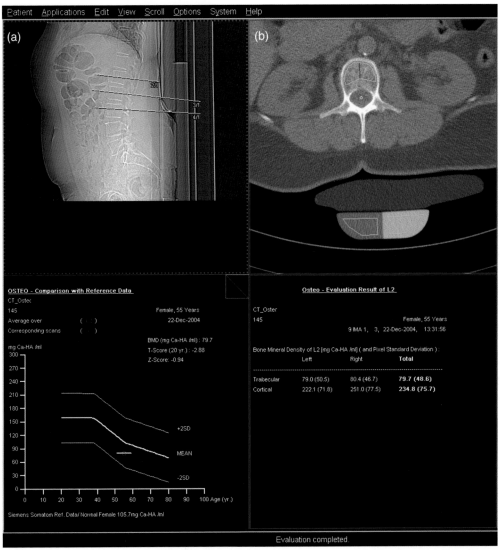

Figure 5.18 (a) Lateral quantitative computed tomography (QCT) showing midpoint identification L1–L3 vertebrae. (b) Transverse QCT at the midpoint showing normal bone density for cortical and trabecular bone. Courtesy of Drs Kroll and Winter, Siemens AG, Berlin

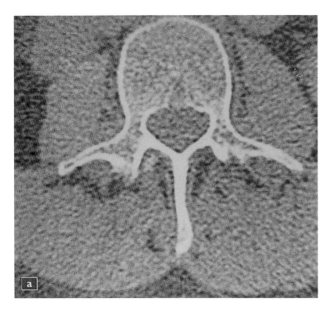

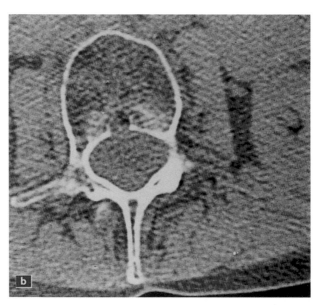

Figure 5.19 Transverse QCT (Siemens Somatom Plus 2) of lumbar vertebrae in a normal subject (a) and a patient with osteoporosis (b). The clear distinction between outer cortical and inner trabecular bone enables measurement of each component. Courtesy of Ms Linda Banks

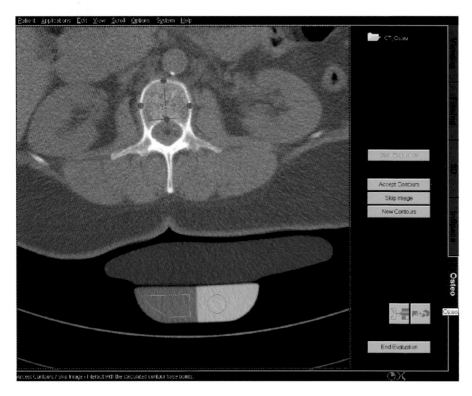

Figure 5.20 An enlarged view of Figure 5.18b shows clear differentiation of cortical from trabecular bone. Courtesy of Drs Kroll and Winter, Siemens AG, Berlin

Dual-energy scanning (with double the radiation dose) may improve the accuracy, but worsen the precision. The radiation dose (200 mrem per single-energy vertebral body scan[21]) and cost are considerably greater than with the methods described above. An advantage of CT is that trabecular bone is distinguished from cortical bone (Figure 5.20), and extraosseous calcium, which artificially increases the bone density measured by DEXA, is readily identified (Figures 5.21 and 5.22)[22]. Trabecular diameter and intertrabecular spaces can be measured using high-resolution CT, and abnormal trabecular architecture can be identified[23]. The recent development of

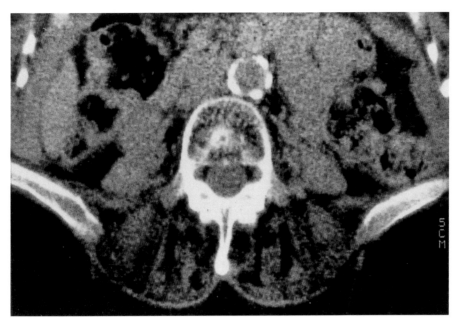

Figure 5.21 Transverse QCT (Siemens Somatom Plus) showing aortic calcification and an intravertebral sclerotic area, both of which affect dual-photon absorptiometry (DPA) and DEXA measurements. Courtesy of Ms Linda Banks

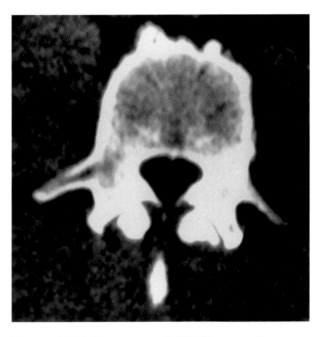

Figure 5.22 Transverse QCT (Siemens Somatom Plus) showing extraneous calcification in the vertebral cortex due to degenerative changes, which affects DPA and DEXA measurements. Courtesy of Ms Linda Banks

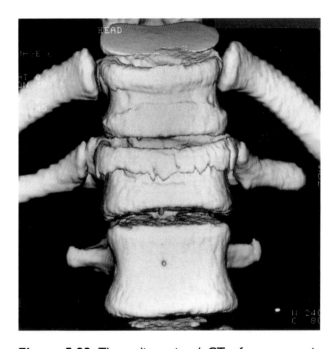

Figure 5.23 Three-dimensional CT of osteoporotic vertebral crush fractures (anteroposterior view). Courtesy of Siemens AG, Erlangen, Germany

three-dimensional (3-D) CT (Figures 5.23 and 5.24) allows assessment of 3-D trabecular structural characteristics and may improve the ability to understand the pathophysiology of osteoporosis, to test the efficacy of pharmaceutical intervention, and to estimate bone biomechanical properties[24].

NUCLEAR MAGNETIC RESONANCE SCANNING

Reports of magnetic resonance imaging of the radius indicate that density measurements correlate well with trabecular bone mineral density as measured by CT[14], and that imaging of the spine using nuclear magnetic resonance can distinguish

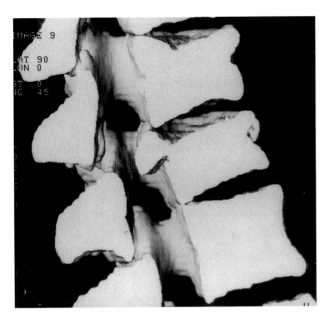

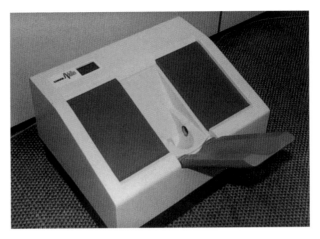

Figure 5.25 Apparatus (Lunar Achilles) for ultrasound measurement of the calcaneus. Courtesy of GE Lunar, Madison, WI

Figure 5.24 Three-dimensional CT of osteoporotic vertebral crush fractures (lateral view). Courtesy of Siemens AG, Erlangen, Germany

osteoporotics and non-osteoporotics[25,26]. Different nuclear magnetic resonance imaging techniques are currently under further investigation, including proximal femoral[27] and distal radius[28] bone structure measurement.

ULTRASONOGRAPHY

The attenuation of ultrasound signals during their passage through bone may be measured by determining the reduction in ultrasound signal amplitude. Several ultrasound parameters used to characterize bone have been proposed, including broadband ultrasound attenuation (BUA), speed of sound (SOS), combined index, amplitude-dependent speed of sound (AD-SoS) and others. Broadband ultrasonic attenuation describes the increase in ultrasound attenuation over a particular frequency range, typically 0.2–0.6 MHz, and may be used to estimate bone mineral density of the calcaneus (Figure 5.25)[29]. The heel is placed in a small water bath between two ultrasonic transducers at a fixed separation. One transducer acts as a transmitter, the other as a receiver. The measurement takes between 1 and 10 min, depending on the type of machinery, and involves

no ionizing radiation. The velocity of ultrasound through the heel can also be measured[30]. Other systems do not require the use of a water bath.

Several studies have shown significant correlations between calcaneus broadband ultrasonic attenuation and spine or hip bone mineral density as measured by DEXA[31] or dual-photon absorptiometry (DPA)[32–34], although one report found a poor relationship between broadband ultrasonic attenuation and DEXA measurements of the spine and hip[35]. Wasnich and colleagues[36] reported that calcaneus bone mineral density (measured by SPA) was as effective as lumbar spine or radius bone mineral density in predicting fracture. A study[37] of 4698 women aged 69 years or more reported that the broadband ultrasonic attenuation at the calcaneus is related to the incidence of past fracture of the hip, and that this relationship is partly independent of bone mineral density.

Ultrasound instruments have theoretical advantages over DEXA in that they are radiation-free, portable, and inexpensive. However, at present, clinical use of ultrasound is difficult because of the absence of clear diagnostic criteria and the use of a variety of instruments. Because of the technological differences between devices, results cannot be extrapolated from one device to another[38].

A T score threshold of −2.5 is probably inappropriate for the diagnosis of osteoporosis by quantitative ultrasound (QUS). A recent study demonstrated that a T score of −1.8 for calcaneal US resulted in the same percentage of postmenopausal women classified as osteoporotic as a T-score <−2.5 for BMD measurements[39].

A report of equivalent T score thresholds for ultrasound measurements at tibia, radius, phalanx, and metatarsal in 278 healthy premenopausal women, 194 postmenopausal women, and 115 women with vertebral fracture demonstrated different T score cut-off values for each skeletal site measured by QUS[40].

Using a combination of both bone mineral density and broadband ultrasonic attenuation measurements may prove to have higher sensitivity and specificity for predicting fracture risk than the use of each method alone.

REFERENCES

1. World Health Organization. Assessment of fracture risk and its application to screening for postmenopausal osteoporosis. World Health Organization Technical Report Series. Geneva: WHO, 1994.

2. Siris ES, Miller PD, Barrett-Connor E et al. Identification and fracture outcomes of undiagnosed low bone mineral density in postmenopausal women. JAMA 2001; 286: 2815–22.

3. Pasco JA, Seeman E, Henry MJ et al. The population burden of fractures originates in women with osteopenia, not osteoporosis. Osteoporos Int 2006; 17: 1404–9.

4. Stulberg BN, Bauer TW, Watson JT, Richmond B. Bone quality. Roentgenographic versus histologic assessment of hip bone structure. Clin Orthop 1989; 240: 200–5.

5. Hurxthal LM, Vose GP, Dotter WE. Densitometric and visual observations of spinal radiographs. Geriatrics 1969; 24: 93–106.

6. Stevenson JC, Banks LM, Spinks TJ et al. Regional and total skeletal measurements in the early postmenopause. J Clin Invest 1987; 80: 258–62.

7. Doyle FH. Involutional osteoporosis. In: MacIntyre I, ed. Clinics in Endocrinology and Metabolism. London: WB Saunders, 1972: 143–67.

8. Grubb SA, Jacobson PC, Aubrey BJ et al. Bone density in osteoporotic women: a modified distal radius density measurement procedure to develop an 'at risk' value for use in screening women. J Orthop Res 1984; 2: 328–32.

9. Chrischilles E, Shireman T, Wallace R. Costs and health effects of osteoporotic fractures. Bone 1994; 15: 377–86.

10. Borg J, Mollgaard A, Riis BJ. Single x-ray absorptiometry: performance characteristics and comparison with single-photon absorptiometry. Osteoporos Int 1995; 5: 377–81.

11. Banks LM, Stevenson JC. Developments in computerized axial tomography scanning and its use in bone disease measurement. In: Stevenson J, ed. New Techniques in Metabolic Bone Disease. London: Wright, 1990:138–56.

12. Lindsay R. Pathogenesis, detection and prevention of postmenopausal osteoporosis. In: Studd J, Whitehead M, eds. The Menopause. Oxford: Blackwell Scientific Publications, 1988: 156–67.

13. Guglielmi G, Grimston SK, Fischer KC, Pacifici R. Osteoporosis: diagnosis with lateral and posteroanterior dual x-ray absorptiometry compared with quantitative CT. Radiology 1994; 192: 845–50.

14. Jergas M, Breitenseher M, Gluer CC et al. Estimates of volumetric bone density from projectional measurements improve the discriminatory capability of dual x-ray absorptiometry. J Bone Miner Res 1995; 10: 1101–10.

15. Briggs AM, Wark JD, Kantor S et al. In vivo intra-operator and inter-operator precision of measuring apparent bone mineral density in vertebral subregions using supine lateral dual-energy x-ray absorptiometry. J Clin Densitom 2005; 8: 314–19.

16. Hamdy RC, Petak SM, Lenchik L; International Society for Clinical Densitometry Position Development Panel and Scientific Advisory Committee. Which central dual X-ray absorptiometry skeletal sites and regions of interest should be used to determine the diagnosis of osteoporosis? J Clin Densitom 2002; 5 (Suppl): S11–18.

17. Grampp S, Jergas M, Lang P et al. Quantitative CT assessment of the lumbar spine and radius in patients with osteoporosis. Am J Roentgenol 1996; 167: 133–40.

18. Grampp S, Lang P, Jergas M et al. Assessment of the skeletal status by peripheral quantitative computed tomography of the forearm: short-term precision in vivo and comparison to dual

x-ray absorptiometry. J Bone Miner Res 1995; 10: 1566–76.

19. Clowes JA, Eastell R, Peel NF. The discriminative ability of peripheral and axial bone measurements to identify proximal femoral, vertebral, distal forearm and proximal humeral fractures: a case control study. Osteoporos Int 2005; 16: 1794–802.

20. Milos G, Spindler A, Ruegsegger P et al. Cortical and trabecular bone density and structure in anorexia nervosa. Osteoporos Int 2005; 16: 783–90.

21. Banks LM, Stevenson JC. Modified method of spinal computed tomography for trabecular bone mineral measurements. J Comput Assist Tomogr 1986; 10: 463–7.

22. Sandor T, Felsenberg D, Kalender WA et al. Compact and trabecular components of the spine using quantitative computed tomography. Calcif Tissue Int 1992; 50: 502–6.

23. Mundinger A, Wiesmeier B, Dinkel E et al. Quantitative image analysis of vertebral body architecture – improved diagnosis in osteoporosis based on high-resolution computed tomography. Br J Radiol 1993; 66: 209–13.

24. Jiang Y, Zhao J, Liao EY et al. Application of micro-CT assessment of 3-D bone microstructure in preclinical and clinical studies. J Bone Miner Metab 2005; 23 (Suppl): 122–31.

25. Wehrli FW, Ford JC, Haddad JG. Osteoporosis: clinical assessment with quantitative MR imaging in diagnosis. Radiology 1995; 196: 631–41.

26. Schick F, Seitz D, Machann J et al. Magnetic resonance bone densitometry. Comparison of different methods based on susceptibility. Invest Radiol 1995; 30: 254–65.

27. Krug R, Banerjee S, Han ET et al. Feasibility of in vivo structural analysis of high-resolution magnetic resonance images of the proximal femur. Osteoporos Int 2005; 16: 1307–14.

28. Hudelmaier M, Kollstedt A, Lochmuller EM et al. Gender differences in trabecular bone architecture of the distal radius assessed with magnetic resonance imaging and implications for mechanical competence. Osteoporos Int 2005; 16: 1124–33.

29. Langton CM, Palmer SB, Porter RW. The measurement of broadband ultrasonic attenuation in cancellous bone. N Engl J Med 1984; 13: 89–91.

30. Herd RJ, Ramalingham T, Ryan PJ et al. Measurements of broadband ultrasonic attenuation in the calcaneus in premenopausal and postmenopausal women. Osteoporos Int 1992; 2: 247–51.

31. Argen M, Karellas A, Leahey D et al. Ultrasound attenuation of the calcaneus: a sensitive and specific discriminator of osteopenia in postmenopausal women. Calcif Tissue Int 1991; 48: 240–4.

32. Rossman P, Zagzebski J, Mesina C et al. Comparison of speed of sound and ultrasound attenuation in the os calcis to bone density of the radius, femur and lumbar spine. Clin Phys Physiol Meas 1989; 10: 353–60.

33. McCloskey EV, Murray SA, Miller C et al. Broadband ultrasound attenuation in the os calcis: relationship to bone mineral at other skeletal sites. Clin Sci 1990; 78: 227–33.

34. Baran DT, Kelly AM, Karella A et al. Ultrasound attenuation of the os calcis in women with osteoporosis and hip fractures. Calcif Tissue Int 1988; 43: 138–42.

35. Massie A, Reid DM, Porter RW. Screening for osteoporosis: comparison between dual-energy x-ray absorptiometry and broadband ultrasound attenuation in 1000 perimenopausal women. Osteoporos Int 1993; 3: 107–10.

36. Wasnich RD, Ross PD, Hellbrun LK, Vogel JM. Prediction of postmenopausal fracture risk with use of bone mineral measurements. Am J Obstet Gynecol 1985; 153: 745–51.

37. Gluer CC, Cummings SR, Bauer DC et al. Osteoporosis: ssociation of recent fractures with quantitative US findings. Radiology 1996; 199: 725–32.

38. Glüer CC, Eastell R, Reid DM et al. Association of five quantitative ultrasound devices and bone densitometry with osteoporotic vertebral fractures in population-based sample: the OPUS study. J Bone Miner Res 2004; 19: 782–93.

39. Frost ML, Blake GM, Fogelman I. Can the WHO criteria for diagnosing osteoporosis be applied to calcaneal quantitative ultrasound? Osteoporos Int 2000; 11: 321–30.

40. Knapp KM, Blake GM, Spector TD et al. Can the WHO definition of osteoporosis be applied to multi-site axial transmission quantitative ultrasound? Osteoporos Int 2004; 15: 367–74.

CHAPTER 6

Management

GENERAL MANAGEMENT AND INVESTIGATION

Although most women presenting with osteoporosis in the postmenopausal period will not have a secondary cause for their low bone mineral density (BMD) it is important not to forget that in some women there will be an illness or medication causing their osteoporosis (Tables 6.1 and 6.2), and efforts should be made to treat such conditions or change relevant medication, when possible.

Important secondary causes of osteoporosis which may be missed include primary hyperparathyroidism and hyperthyroidism, either of which may decrease bone density by 10–20%, and these conditions and others should be sought from the medical history, physical examination, and appropriate investigation (Table 6.1). Serum 25-hydroxyvitamin D (25-OHD) and parathyroid hormone measurements can be used to exclude vitamin D deficiency and secondary hyperparathyroididsm in, for example, patients with limited sunlight exposure or malabsorption, or in those using anticonvulsant treatment. Baseline serum 25-OHD and parathyroid hormone measurements may be performed even if calcium and vitamin D supplementation is planned, as they can be repeated to ensure an adequate response to treatment.

DRUG TREATMENT

The methods of drug treatment of osteoporosis may be broadly divided into those that retard bone resorption, such as estrogens, calcitonin,

and bisphosphonates, and those that stimulate bone formation, such as teriparatide and strontium ranelate (which also has some antiresorptive activity). Antiresorptive agents decrease bone resorption and, due to transient uncoupling of bone turnover, result in a small increase in BMD of between 5 and 10%, usually in the first or second year of treatment. In contrast, anabolic agents can increase BMD by up to 20%. Recently, combined regimens have been under investigation

HORMONE REPLACEMENT THERAPY

Estrogen therapy is a commonly used prophylactic measure, and has been shown to reduce the frequency of osteoporotic fracture. Until recently, few prospective studies of the effect of hormone replacement theraphy (HRT) on fracture risk had been published. In a report of 3140 peri- and postmenopausal women followed for a mean of 2.5 years, the age-adjusted risk of fracture was 0.75 (95% confidence interval (CI) 0.5–0.96) for HRT users compared with non-users[1]. Several retrospective studies have shown that the use of estrogens for 5 years is associated with a 50% reduction in the risk of hip fracture[2–4] and a reduced rate of vertebral fracture[5]. Estrogens may reduce the rate of fracture by increasing mobility and dexterity, but the majority of their effect is likely to be due to their action on bone density and turnover. In addition, recent evidence shows that estrogen may maintain vertebral disc height, and hence shock-absorbing capacity, which may also help to reduce vertebral fracture[6].

Table 6.1 Secondary causes of osteoporosis: diseases and investigations

Disease	Laboratory investigations
Endocrine disorders	
• hyperparathyroidism	Calcium, phosphate, alkaline phosphatase, PTH, 25 hydroxyvitamin D, kidney function
• hyperthyroidism	TSH, free T_4, free T_3
• hypercortisolism	Cortisol, ACTH, dexamethasone suppression
• hypogonadism	Estradiol, FSH, LH, testosterone, SHBG
• prolactinoma	Prolactin
• diabetes mellitus (type I)	Fasting glucose, glucose tolerance, glycated Hb
Connective tissue disorders	
• rheumatoid arthritis	ESR, rheumatoid factor, antinuclear antibodies
• osteogenesis imperfecta	
• Marfan's syndrome	
• Ehlers-Danlos syndrome	
Reticulo-endothelial disorders	
• Leukemia	Full blood count, ESR
• Hodgkins disease	
• non-Hodgkins lymphoma	
Metastatic carcinoma	
Multiple myeloma	Serum protein electrophoresis, urinary Bence-Jones protein
Respiratory diseases	
• cystic fibrosis	
• chronic obstructive pulmonary disease	
• diffuse parenchymal lung disease	
• primary pulmonary hypertension	
Liver diseases	
• primary biliary cirrhosis	Liver function
Anorexia nervosa	
Mastocytosis	Urine histamine/prostaglandin D2
Thalassemia	Full blood count, hemoglobin electrophoresis

Table 6.2 Other secondary causes of osteoporosis

Drugs
- corticosteroids
- anticonvulsants (osteomalacia)
- thyroxine (excess)
- GnRH agonists
- aromatase inhibitors
- cytotoxic agents
- heparin
- rosiglitazone
- Selective serotonin re-uptake inhibitors

Immobilization/weightlessness
Juvenile
Pregnancy-induced
Idiopathic

Many prospective controlled studies of the effects of estrogen on bone density have been conducted. The study by Lindsay and Hart[7] was one of the earliest reports, and measured metacarpal density, using single-photon absorptiometry (SPA) of the metacarpal, in 120 postmenopausal women who were randomized to one of four groups taking different dosages of conjugated equine estrogen and a control group. There was no reduction in mean bone density in women taking 0.625 mg/day and 1.25 mg/day over 2 years, but there was a mean fall in density of 5% and 8% in the two groups of women taking 0.3 mg/day and 0.15 mg/day, respectively, and a fall of 8% in the controls. Christiansen and co-workers[8] used SPA to examine the changes in forearm bone density over 1 year in 69 early-postmenopausal women randomized to three different dosages of oral estradiol and a control group. Bone density in the control group fell by 2%, but rose by 1.5% and 0.8% in those women taking 4 mg/day and 2 mg/day of estradiol, respectively, and did not change in those taking 1 mg/day.

Whilst a dose-dependent effect of estrogen has been shown in several studies, it has also been found that older postmenopausal women may not need as much estrogen as younger women to achieve the same skeletal effect. Lees and Stevenson[9] conducted a double-blind, randomized, placebo-controlled study of the effects of two different doses (1 mg and 2 mg) of oral estradiol with the cyclical addition of various doses of dydrogesterone. Spinal and hip bone density was measured by dual-energy X-ray absorptiometry (DEXA) for 2 years. The bone density rose in all treated groups, with a somewhat greater increase with the higher dose, and fell in the placebo group. The increase in spine bone density for the 1-mg estradiol group in the oldest quartile of women was similar to that seen with 2 mg estradiol in the youngest quartile of women (Figure 6.1).

The estrogen plus progestin component of the Women's Health Initiative[10] provided the first robust placebo-controlled data concerning the effects of HRT on fracture risk. This was a randomized controlled primary-prevention trial (planned duration 8.5 years) in which 16 608 postmenopausal women aged 50–79 years with an intact uterus at baseline were recruited by 40 US clinical centers in 1993–1998 and randomized to receive conjugated equine estrogens, 0.625 mg/day, plus medroxyprogesterone acetate, 2.5 mg/day, in one tablet ($n = 8506$), or placebo ($n = 8102$). The hazard ratio (CI) for hip fracture was 0.66 (0.45–0.98), for vertebral fracture was 0.66 (0.44–0.98), and was 0.76 (0.69–0.85) for combined fractures (Figure 6.2). The absolute reduced risk per 10 000 person-years attributable to estrogen plus progestin was five fewer hip fractures.

The estrogen-alone component of the Women's Health Initiative[11] enrolled 10 739 postmenopausal women aged 50–79 years with prior hysterectomy, including 23% of minority race/ethnicity, who were randomly assigned to receive either 0.625 mg/day of conjugated equine estrogen or placebo. The estimated hazard ratio for hip fracture was 0.61 (0.41–0.91) and for all fractures was 0.70 (0.63–0.79). The study reported an absolute risk reduction of six fewer hip fractures per 10 000 person-years.

Estradiol implants appear to preserve bone density. McKay Hart and colleagues[12] followed up 19 oophorectomized women treated with 50-mg estradiol implants every 6 months for 2 years. The bone mineral density in the lumbar spine (measured by dual-photon absorptiometry (DPA)) increased by 4.3% per year. A similar increase of

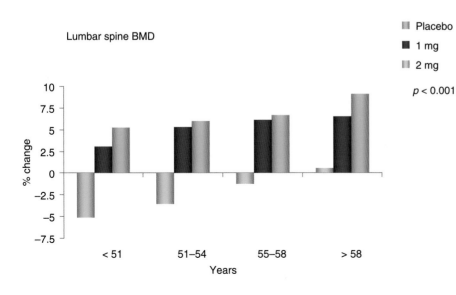

Figure 6.1 Percentage changes in vertebral bone mineral density (BMD) in response to two doses of estrogen according to age quartiles. From reference 9, with permission

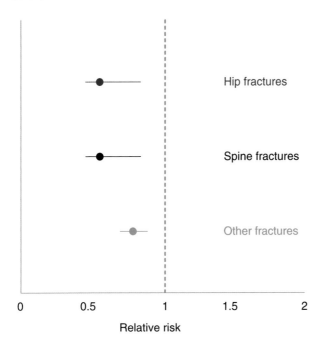

0   0.5   1   1.5   2

Relative risk

Figure 6.2 Relative risk of spine, hip, or other fractures with hormone replacement therapy (HRT) compared with placebo. The Women's Health Initiative. From reference 10, with permission

3.3% per year in trabecular bone density (measured by computed tomography (CT)) has been reported over a 3-year period with the same treatment regimen[13]. The results of a cross-sectional study comparing the effects of oral estrogens and implant estradiol and testosterone therapy on spine and femoral bone density suggested a greater rise in bone mineral density in women treated with implants[14]. The bone mineral density increases with implant therapy appear to be highest in women who have the highest estradiol levels during treatment[15].

Transdermal estrogen therapy appears to produce similar effects to oral therapy. Riis and co-workers[16] found increases in bone mineral density in the spine in postmenopausal women treated with percutaneous estradiol combined with oral progesterone. In a study of spine and hip bone density (using DPA) in 66 postmenopausal women randomized to receive either transdermal HRT (estradiol-17β at 0.05 mg daily with norethisterone acetate at 0.25 mg daily for 14 of every 28 days) or oral therapy (continuous equine estrogen at 0.625 mg daily with DL-norgestrel at 0.15 mg

daily for 12 of every 28 days), and compared with a reference group studied concurrently[17], bone mineral density was measured at 6-month intervals for 3 years, and skeletal turnover was assessed by serum measurements of calcium, phosphate, and alkaline phosphatase, and by urine estimations of hydroxyproline/creatinine and calcium/creatinine excretion. Vertebral and femoral bone mineral density rose significantly in both treatment groups and fell in the reference group (Figures 6.3 and 6.4). The biochemical measurements indicated a significant reduction in bone turnover in the treated groups.

Several studies suggest that a small proportion of women taking estrogen at currently accepted 'bone-preserving' doses will not maintain their bone mineral density. This may be due to variations in the absorption of estrogen, failure of compliance, or individual differences in the response of bone to estrogen. Unfortunately, the literature so far does not allow any firm conclusions to be drawn, as the designs of many of the studies showing loss of bone mineral density with standard doses of estrogen do not include sufficient data on compliance or estrogen levels[5,18]. Spinal bone density was not maintained in one-third of oophorectomized women treated with 0.625 mg/day of conjugated equine estrogen[5] and in 22% of women following a natural menopause[18]. It has been demonstrated that 12% of women taking either estradiol-17β at 0.05 mg/day with norethisterone acetate 0.25 mg/day for 14 of every 28 days or continuous equine estrogen at 0.625 mg/day with DL-norgestrel at 0.15 mg/day for 12 of every 28 days with good compliance for 3 years will show significant loss of bone in the proximal femur[17].

Withdrawal of estrogen treatment appears to result in bone loss at a rate similar to that in the immediate postmenopausal period[19,20]; thus, it has been suggested that the effect of estrogen on bone mineral density is to 'buy time'[21]. In women who discontinue treatment, the amount of bone 'bought' is probably the duration of estrogen use multiplied by the rate of bone loss duri`ng the slow phase (approximately 1% per year) after the period of fast loss in the early postmenopausal years (Figure 6.5).

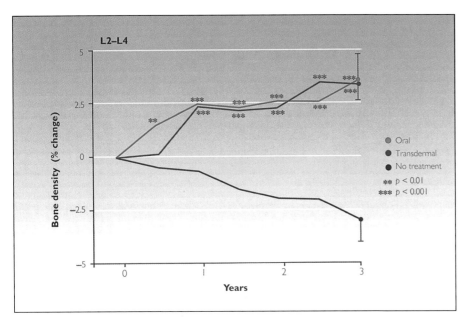

Figure 6.3 Changes in spine (L2-L4) bone density with oral and transdermal estrogen therapy compared with no estrogen treatment. From reference 17, with permission

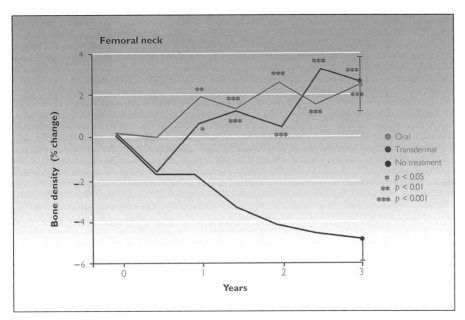

Figure 6.4 Changes in femoral neck bone density with oral and transdermal estrogen therapy compared with no estrogen treatment. From reference 17, with permission

But HRT use in the early postmenopause may still result in fracture reduction in later years. Women who participated in randomized clinical trials with HRT or placebo were followed subsequently without further treatment for up to 15 years[22]. Those who had been randomized to take HRT had a significantly reduced fracture risk compared to those randomized to placebo (Figure 6.6). One report demonstrated that estrogen was most effective in preventing hip fractures in women over 75 years of age[23]. It has been suggested that an effective strategy to prevent fracture in postmenopausal women would be to target elderly women with a high risk of osteoporotic fracture, in whom short periods of treatment appear to have profound effects on fracture risk[24]. In support of this, it has been shown[25] that the administration of unopposed very low dose transdermal estradiol (14 μg daily) will conserve bone density in elderly women with osteoporosis whilst having minimal endometrial effects or other side-effects.

The mechanism of the effect of estrogens on bone is uncertain, and is discussed in more detail in Chapter 2. Estrogens may have a direct effect on osteoblasts or on the cytokines that regulate osteoblast formation such as interleukin-1 (IL-1)

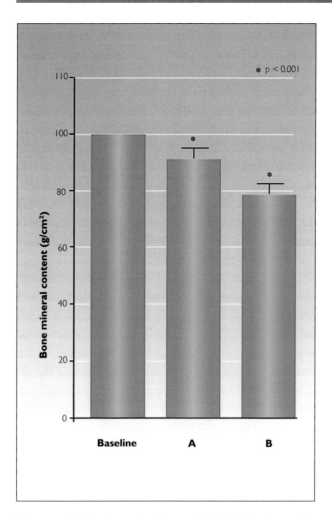

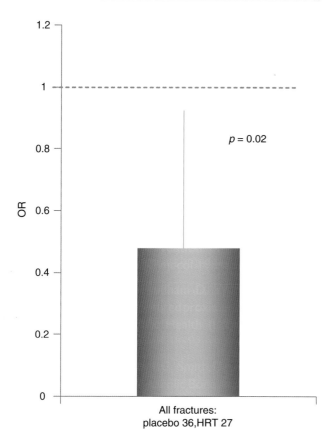

Figure 6.6 Odds ratio (OR) for fracture in women who had been randomized to HRT compared with placebo. The PERF study. From reference 22, with permission

Figure 6.5 Prolonged effect of HRT following withdrawal of treatment. Bone density, as measured by single-photon absorptiometry (SPA) in the distal radius, is expressed as the initial percentage value (±SEM) in 242 healthy postmenopausal women at baseline and after 12 years. Group A (n = 68) received HRT for a mean of 5.4 years followed by a period off treatment; group B (n = 177) received no treatment for 12 years. *p < 0.001. From reference 21, with permission

or tumor necrosis factor (TNF). They may also have an indirect effect on bone by increasing calcitonin secretion or by influencing local factors. It has been suggested that, although HRT increases bone mineral density, it may not have an effect on trabecular architecture, and is unable to reverse structural disruption in women with postmenopausal osteoporosis[26].

In summary, HRT is an effective treatment for the prevention of vertebral and non-vertebral fractures, and many maintain that HRT should remain first-line treatment for this indication, since other currently available treatments are not as effective in this respect[27]. Meta-analyses have reported a 33% reduction in vertebral fracture and a 27% reduction in non-vertebral fracture with HRT use[28,29], but an attenuated effect with age. However, more recent findings suggest that just a few years' treatment with HRT around the time of the menopause may result in lasting skeletal benefit in terms of fracture reduction in later years[22], and that the use of unopposed ultra-low dose estrogen may be an effective treatment for elderly women with osteoporosis[25].

SELECTIVE ESTROGEN RECEPTOR MODULATORS

Concerns regarding the long-term effects of estrogen on the risk of breast cancer and on the endometrium have led to the development of selective estrogen receptor modulators (SERMs). Raloxifene is a non-steroidal benzothiophene that inhibits bone mineral density loss, but does not stimulate the endometrium and is an estrogen antagonist for breast tissue. It does not appear to be a useful treatment for climacteric hot flushes.

In a 2-year multicenter, placebo-controlled, double-blind study, Delmas and co-workers[30] randomized 661 postmenopausal women to receive 30, 60, or 150 mg of raloxifene per day or placebo. Of these women, 55% had low bone mineral density. The densities of the hip and spine were measured by DEXA every 6 months. Biochemical markers of bone turnover were measured every 3 months and included serum osteocalcin, serum bone-specific alkaline phosphatase, and the urinary type I collagen C-telopeptide-to-creatinine ratio. By the end of the study, 25% of the participants had dropped out.

Bone mineral density increased significantly in the lumbar spine, total hip, femoral neck, and total body in all three treatment groups, and fell in the placebo group (Figures 6.7 and 6.8). The increase in bone mineral density at most sites was greatest in the group that received raloxifene 150 mg/day although, in the total hip, the greatest increase was seen in the 60-mg/day group. Compared with placebo, each of the treatments statistically significantly decreased concentrations of the three markers of bone turnover (Figure 6.9).

In the MORE (Multiple Outcomes of Raloxifene Evaluation) study of 7705 postmenopausal osteoporotic women aged 31–80 years, raloxifene increased lumbar spine and femoral neck BMD by 2–3%, reduced the risk of vertebral fractures by 30–50%, and decreased the incidence of breast cancer[31,32]. The RUTH (Raloxifene Use for The Heart) study[33] of over 10 000 women confirmed the reduction in vertebral fractures, and the reduction of breast cancer, but demonstrated conclusively that raloxifene does not reduce hip fracture incidence (Figure 6.10). Thus, raloxifene can be used for the prevention of vertebral fractures in women with osteopenia/osteoporosis, but its use is not appropriate for women who are at high risk of non-vertebral fractures.

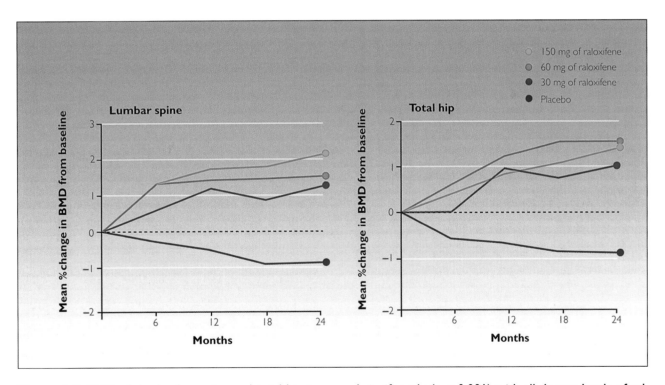

Figure 6.7 BMD of the lumbar spine and total hip increased significantly (*p* < 0.001) with all dosage levels of raloxifene. From reference 30, with permission

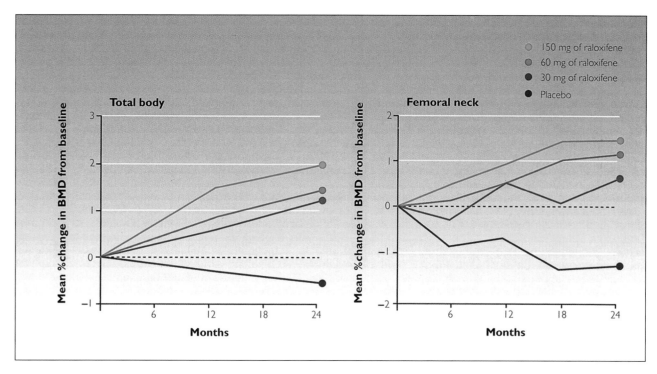

Figure 6.8 BMD of the femoral neck and total body increased significantly ($p < 0.001$) with all dosage levels of raloxifene. From reference 30, with permission

CALCITONIN

Calcitonin directly suppresses the activity of osteoclasts and also inhibits their recruitment (Figure 6.11). It has been isolated from a large number of animal species. Calcitonin from fish is the most resistant to degradation in humans and, thus, has the greatest potency per unit weight. It is not yet known whether calcitonins from other species will be more effective. Daily intramuscular salmon calcitonin at a relatively high dosage (100 IU) has been shown to prevent bone loss and slightly increase skeletal mass in women with osteoporotic fractures[35]. In healthy women, a much lower dose (20 IU) of synthetic human calcitonin, given subcutaneously three times a week in the early postmenopausal period, was as effective as estrogen in preventing spinal trabecular bone loss[36]. The inconvenience of injectable calcitonin led to the development of alternative methods of administration. Reports of the use of salmon calcitonin suppositories have failed to show effects on spinal or femoral bone mineral density, or on markers of bone turnover[37], and the suppositories are reported to have poor tolerability[38]. However,

studies of intranasal salmon calcitonin suggest that it may be of value in both the prevention and treatment of osteoporosis[39–44].

In a double-blind, placebo-controlled trial[45], the effects of intranasal salmon calcitonin on bone mineral density were studied for 2 years in 117 postmenopausal women with reduced bone density. The subjects were randomized to receive salmon calcitonin 200 IU daily or three times a week, or placebo. Compared with placebo, daily salmon calcitonin resulted in no significant loss in lumbar bone mineral density over 2 years (Figure 6.12). In this group of women, those who were more than 5 years past the menopause showed the greatest response. Although there was no difference in changes in proximal femoral bone density among the three groups, bone mineral density did not fall significantly in women taking daily salmon calcitonin. Significant bone loss in both the spine and proximal femur was seen in women receiving thrice-weekly salmon calcitonin or placebo. There were no significant treatment-related adverse effects and salmon calcitonin was well tolerated.

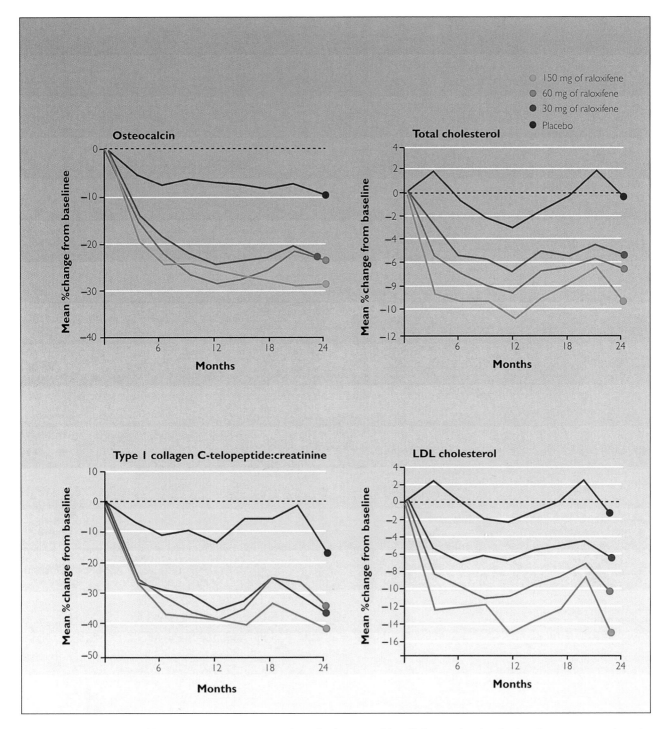

Figure 6.9 Markers of bone turnover were significantly decreased by all dosage levels of raloxifene compared to the placebo group as were total and low-density lipoprotein (LDL) cholesterol. From reference 30, with permission

A 5-year, double-blind, randomized, placebo-controlled study of the effects of calcitonin nasal spray on vertebral fracture comprised 1255 postmenopausal women[46] with established osteoporosis who were randomized to placebo, or 100, 200, or 400 IU/day of nasal spray. A 36% reduction in risk of new vertebral fracture was observed in women taking 200 IU/day (relative risk 0.64, 95% CI 0.47–0.97, $p = 0.03$). Although the PROOF (Prevent Recurrence of Osteoporotic Fractures) study[47] demonstrated that intranasal salmon calcitonin 200 IU daily appeared effective and safe for the prevention of bone loss in postmenopausal women with reduced bone mass,

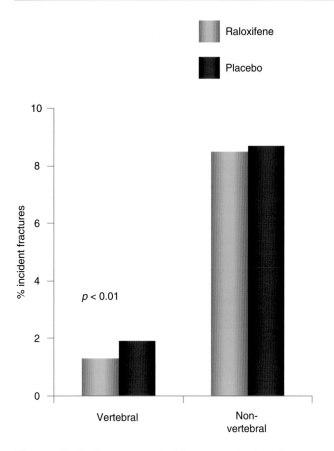

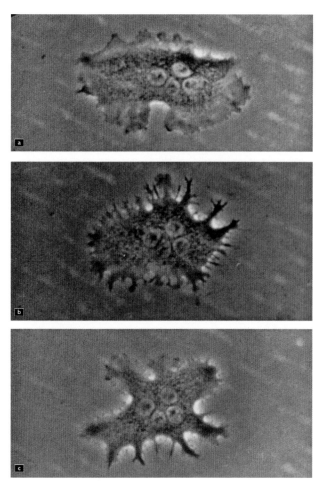

Figure 6.10 Percentage incident vertebral and non-vertebral fractures with either raloxifene or placebo. The RUTH study. From reference 33, with permission

Figure 6.11 Time-lapse sequence of scanning electron micrographs shows the response of an isolated osteoclast to calcitonin at time 0 (a), 10 min (b), and 120 min (c). From reference 34, with permission

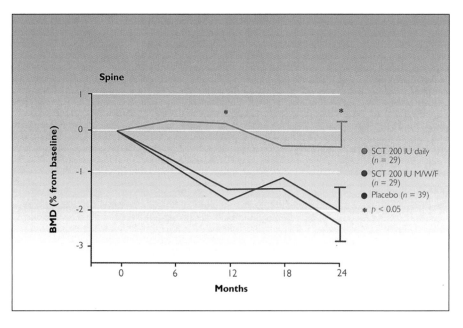

Figure 6.12 Percentage changes in spine BMD with salmon calcitonin (SCT) 200 IU daily compared with 200 IU three times a week and placebo over 2 years. From reference 45, with permission

decreases in fractures with 100 and 400 IU were not statistically significant. A review of 14 trials of parenteral and intranasal calcitonin involving a total of 1309 men and women showed a 57% reduction in fracture compared with placebo (55% for vertebral and 66% for non-vertebral)[48].

Calcitonin may be useful in the management of the pain associated with acute osteoporotic fractures. In a randomized controlled trial of 100 men and women with acute vertebral crush fractures, 200 IU daily of nasal salmon calcitonin for 28 days decreased pain and resulted in earlier mobilization compared with placebo[49].

BISPHOSPHONATES

Bisphosphonates are stable analogs of pyrophosphate which bind to the bone surface and inhibit osteoclastic activity. As bisphosphonates persist in the skeleton for many months or years, their duration of action is prolonged beyond the period of administration.

Disodium etidronate has been shown to increase bone mineral density in women with spinal osteoporosis compared with placebo-treated controls, who lost bone density[50,51]. The incidence of new fractures in etidronate-treated women in one study[50] was less than that in controls. Etidronate may be of use in the treatment of steroid-induced osteoporosis[52].

There are no interventional studies investigating the effect of etidronate on hip fracture incidence, but epidemiological data suggest that it decreases hip fractures by 44% in women over the age of 76 years[53].

Etidronate has now been superseded by more potent bisphosphonates. In an early study[54], pamidronate given continuously was shown to cause a mean rise in lumbar bone density of approximately 3% per year, although in some patients the bone mineral density increased by 50% after 4 years of treatment. A double-blind placebo-controlled study[55] of 48 postmenopausal women over 2 years indicated that pamidronate 150 mg/day increased the bone mineral density of the lumbar spine, femoral trochanter, and total body.

There have been concerns that continuous use of pamidronate will halt bone remodeling, which will lead to poor microfracture repair and an increase in fracture rate. Intermittent regimens of treatment have been proposed as a method of allowing uncoupling of bone resorption and formation, and intermittent phases of positive bone balance. In a 2-year, prospective, double-blind study[56], 125 women were randomized to receive oral pamidronate 300 mg/day for 4 out of every 12 weeks, oral pamidronate 150 mg/day for 4 out of every 8 weeks, or placebo. Bone mineral density at the lumbar spine and femoral neck increased significantly in the drug-treated women, but declined in women receiving placebo. There were no differences in effect on bone mineral density between the two dose regimens, but withdrawal from the study due to side-effects was nearly three times more common in women receiving the 300-mg/day regimen. In women taking oral pamidronate 150-mg/day for 4 out of every 8 weeks, the drop-out rate because of side-effects was comparable to that with placebo.

Alendronate has been reported to preserve bone mineral density, reduce vertebral and hip fracture risk, and be well tolerated in women with low bone mineral density in large prospective studies[57–59]. In the multicenter, double-blind, 2-year study of Chesnut and co-workers[58], 188 postmenopausal women, aged 42–75 years and with low bone mineral density of the lumbar spine, were randomized to receive placebo or one of five alendronate treatment regimens. Alendronate produced significant reductions in markers of bone resorption and formation, and significantly increased bone mineral density at the lumbar spine, hip, and total body compared with decreases (significant at lumbar spine) in those receiving placebo. The mean changes in bone mineral density over 24 months with alendronate 10 mg were +7% for the lumbar spine, +5% for total hip and +3% for total body (all $p < 0.01$) compared with changes of −1%, −1%, and 0%, respectively, with placebo.

A larger randomized placebo-controlled study of the effects of alendronate on fracture risk in

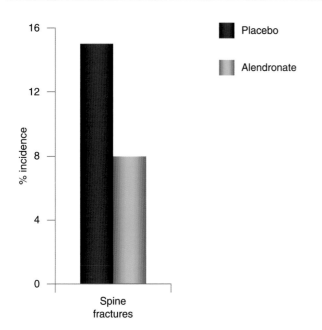

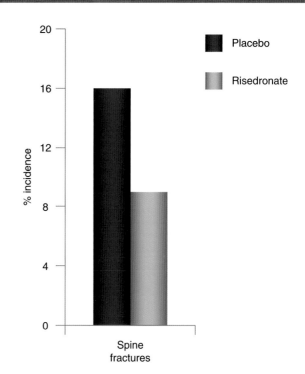

Figure 6.13 Percentage incidence of vertebral fractures in postmenopausal osteoporotic women randomized to alendronate or placebo. The FIT study. From reference 59, with permission

women aged 55–81 years who had at least one vertebral fracture at recruitment (Fracture Intervention Trial Research Group[59]) enrolled a total of 2027 women, randomized to receive either placebo or alendronate (5 mg/day for 2 years followed by 10 mg/day for 1 year). Follow-up radiographs were obtained from 98% of surviving participants (1964 women). The relative risk of one or more new morphometric vertebral fractures for women receiving alendronate was 0.53 (95% CI 0.27–0.72) (Figure 6.13), and the relative risk of hip and wrist fracture was 0.49 (95% CI 0.23–0.99) and 0.52 (95% CI 0.31–0.87), respectively.

Risedronate appears to be effective in the management of postmenopausal osteoporosis[60,61]. The Vertebral Efficacy with Risedronate Therapy Study Group[60,61] reported significant increases in BMD compared with placebo of 5–6% at the lumbar spine, 1.6–3.1% at the femoral neck, and 3.3–6.4% at the femoral trochanter with 3 years treatment. They also reported a 41–49% reduction in the incidence of new vertebral fractures and 33–39% fall in non-vertebral fractures in women treated with risedronate compared with placebo (Figure 6.14).

Figure 6.14 Percentage incidence of vertebral fractures in postmenopausal osteoporotic women randomized to risedronate or placebo. The VERT study. From reference 60, with permission

McClung et al[62] studied 5445 women age 70–79 years with low BMD and 3886 women over 80 years who had at least one clinical risk factor for hip fracture. They were randomized to receive either risedronate or placebo. The incidence of hip fracture in women with low BMD taking risedronate (1.9%) was 40% lower than in those on placebo (3.2%). However, there was no significant reduction in fracture risk with risedronate in the older women (over 80 years).

Newer bisphosphonates

Ibandronate is a potent nitrogen-containing bisphosphonate available as a once-monthly oral formulation for the treatment and prevention of osteoporosis. Preclinical experiments with estrogen-depleted rats, dogs, and monkeys demonstrated the efficacy of daily and intermittent ibandronate dosing[63,64].

In a multinational, double-blind, placebo-controlled, randomized study, oral daily ibandronate (2.5 mg) significantly reduced the risk of new vertebral fractures by 62% relative to placebo after 3 years of treatment, and caused a reduction of 59% in the relative risk of combined new moderate and severe vertebral fractures after 1 year[65]. It has been reported that significantly more women with postmenopausal osteoporosis preferred once-monthly ibandronate therapy to once-weekly alendronate therapy[66].

Zoledronic acid is a newly developed bisphosphonate for the treatment of postmenopausal osteoporosis whose chief advantage is its extended dosing interval. There is evidence of a clinically significant effect on bone density in women with osteoporosis. In a 1-year dose-ranging BMD study in 351 women with postmenopausal osteoporosis, patients who received any of five dosing regimens of intravenous zoledronic acid (0.25 mg every 3 months, 0.5 mg every 3 months, 1 mg every 3 months, 2 mg every 6 months, or 4 mg × 1 dose every 12 months) had significantly (all $p < 0.001$) greater increases in lumbar spine (range 4.3–5.1% higher) and femoral neck (range 3.1–3.5% higher) BMD than patients who received placebo[67]. Musculoskeletal pain (10–20%), fever (9–20%), and arthralgia (8–25%) were common side-effects. A 3-year study of 3889 postmenopausal osteoporotic women given ibandronate 5 mg by short intravenous infusion every 12 months demonstrated a 70% reduction in the risk of morphometric vertebral fractures compared with placebo[68]. Hip fracture risk was reduced by 41%. A more serious side-effect from zoledronate to emerge from this study was an increased risk of atrial fibrillation. Clearly longer-term safety data are still needed.

STRONTIUM RANELATE

Strontium ranelate is an orally active drug that appears to both stimulate bone formation and inhibit bone resorption[69].

The Spinal Osteoporosis Therapeutic Intervention (SOTI) trial of 1649 postmenopausal women with osteoporosis reported a significant 49% reduction in new morphometric vertebral fractures with strontium ranelate 2 g/day relative

to placebo after 1 year, and a significant 41% reduction over 3 years (Figure 6.15)[70].

The Treatment of Peripheral Osteoporosis Study (TROPOS) of 4932 postmenopausal women with osteoporosis reported similar reductions in vertebral fracture risk[71]. In addition, this study reported that treatment with strontium 2 g/day significantly reduced the risk of all non-vertebral fractures by 16% and of major non-vertebral fragility fractures by 19%. The most commonly reported adverse events in the SOTI and TROPOS studies were diarrhea and nausea. In both studies, the differences in diarrhea and nausea between strontium and placebo disappeared after 3 months.

TERIPARATIDE

Teriparatide is the name given to the recombinant parathyroid hormone (PTH). PTH is an 84-amino-acid peptide hormone which is one of the major calcium-regulating hormones. It increases serum calcium by reducing renal excretion and mobilizing bone calcium through increased osteoclastic resorption. It also indirectly

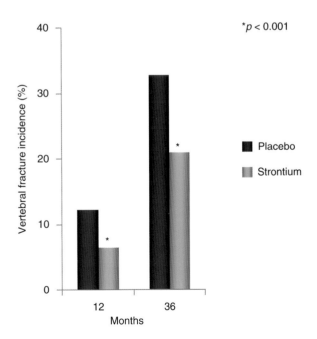

Figure 6.15 Percentage incidence of vertebral fractures in postmenopausal osteoporotic women randomized to strontium ranelate or placebo. The SOTI study. From reference 70, with permission

increases intestinal calcium absorption. However, its effect on bone is also anabolic, and it increases bone formation, as shown by the early studies of Kalu et al[72]. With a continuous administration of parathyroid hormone, such as is seen in primary hyperparathyroidism, bone resorption usually predominates, but when PTH is given intermittently, bone formation predominates. So, in contrast to the antiresorptive agents used to treat osteoporosis, PTH actually increases bone turnover. The biologically active fragment of PTH is the 1–34 amino acid fragment, and this was used in human studies to demonstrate the anabolic effects of the hormone on the skeleton[73,74].

Several clinical studies of teriparatide have shown benefit of the intermittent subcutaneous administration of this peptide on BMD and fracture risk in women with postmenopausal osteoporosis[75–77]. Larger increases in BMD are observed with teriparatide than with other therapies. Importantly, PTH has been shown to improve skeletal architecture, including trabecular connectivity[78,79] (Figure 6.16). Reductions in vertebral fractures of around 65% were reported. Whilst significant reductions in all non-vertebral fractures have been observed, a significant reduction in hip fracture has not yet been established. The concept of combining an anabolic agent with an antiresorptive agent is attractive, and the addition of teriparatide to HRT gave significant improvements in BMD[76]. However, when combined with a bisphosphonate, a blunting of the response to teriparatide has been observed in some[80,81] but not all[82] studies. At present, it seems more prudent to follow teriparatide treatment with bisphosphonates rather than giving them in a combination.

Daily subcutaneous injection of 20 μg teriparatide is approved for the treatment of osteoporosis in postmenopausal women and men, but because of its high cost this is usually confined to those who have severe osteoporosis with a high fracture risk and who are unable to tolerate or respond to other therapies. Teriparatide is usually well tolerated, although it has the drawback of needing to be given by self-administered subcuta-

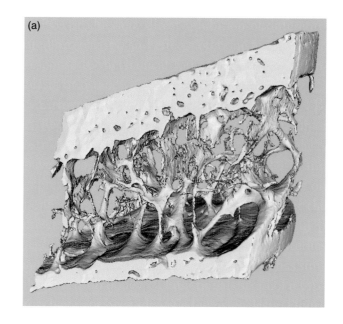

(a)

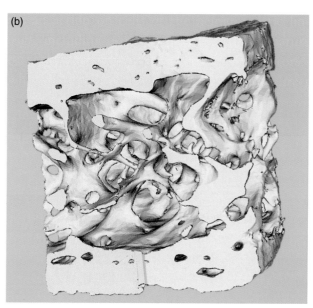

(b)

Figure 6.16 Three-dimensional micro-computed tomography (microCT) reconstructions of paired iliac crest bone biopsies (a) before and (b) after treatment with teriparatide showing increases in cortical thickness, trabecular volume, and connectivity. From reference 79, with permission, courtesy of Eli Lilly & Co, Indianapolis, IN

neous injection. Headache, nausea, and dizziness can occur due to its vasodilatory actions. Mild hypercalcemia and hypercalciuria do not usually cause a problem[75]. Because teriparatide was found to induce osteogenic sarcomas in rats in a dose and duration-dependent manner[83], its use in humans is limited to under 2 years, although no cases of teriparatide-induced osteosarcoma have been reported in humans.

ANABOLIC STEROIDS

It is not known how anabolic steroids produce their effects on bone. It has been postulated that they have a direct effect on osteoblasts or their precursors and/or act to prevent bone resorption. There is evidence *in vitro* for the former effect[84]. It has been suggested that the increase in muscle mass induced by anabolic steroids is partly responsible for increases in bone mineral density[85]. Because of side-effects such as fluid retention and insulin resistance, anabolic steroids are now rarely used for the treatment of osteoporosis.

FLUORIDE

Fluoride appears to stimulate new bone formation, probably by stimulation of proliferation and differentiation of committed osteoblast precursors, or by a direct action on osteoblasts. Several reports show that sodium fluoride is capable of increasing trabecular bone density[86–89], particularly in the spine. However, in one study[87], this was not associated with a reduction in vertebral fracture incidence. There are also reports that fluoride treatment results in an increased incidence of hip fracture[90]. The structural quality of fluoridated hydroxyapatite appears poor (Figure 6.17).

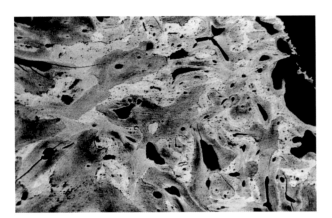

Figure 6.17 Back-scattered electron micrograph of fluorotic bone showing its dense irregular pattern. Courtesy of Professor Alan Boyde

Upper gastrointestinal side-effects may develop in patients taking fluoride, particularly those using non-enteric coated preparations, and approximately 25% of patients develop pseudo-arthritic pains in the joints of the lower limb. Because of these problems, fluoride is rarely used for the treatment of osteoporosis.

VITAMIN D

There is little evidence that vitamin D or its analogs are of any value in the treatment or prevention of osteoporosis for a large proportion of women in Western societies[91–93], although large studies in Japan have shown fracture incidence reduction. However, vitamin D supplementation may be beneficial for elderly or institutionalized vitamin D-deficient women as vitamin D deficiency and secondary hyperparathyroidism are common in such women. A French study of 3270 women (mean age 84 years) living in nursing homes and apartment blocks for the elderly used 800 IU of vitamin D_3 and 1.2 g of elemental calcium daily. This regimen decreased parathyroid hormone levels, increased femoral neck BMD, and reduced the risk of hip fracture by 27%[94]. A study[95] of a Western population using 200 IU of vitamin D for 2 years showed preservation of bone mineral density in the spine, but not in the femoral neck. A recent report[96] from the Women's Health Initiative randomized, controlled trial compared the use of 1000 mg of elemental calcium with 400 IU of vitamin D_3 daily versus placebo in postmenopausal women aged 50–79 years. The follow-up period averaged approximately 7 years. In the active-treatment group, compared with the placebo group, there was a small but statistically significant increase in hip-bone density, but no reduction in the overall rate of hip fracture, which was the primary outcome. Calcium and vitamin D_3 appeared to be well tolerated, but there was an increased risk of kidney stones in women receiving treatment. It is likely that the dosages of vitamin D metabolites necessary to produce a positive effect on bone in women who are not vitamin D deficient are associated with toxicity.

New vitamin D metabolites may avoid such side-effects and studies are awaited with interest.

CALCIUM

It appears that, for the majority of adults following a healthy diet, calcium supplementation has little or no effect on bone mineral density. There have been few satisfactory prospective studies of the effects of calcium supplementation on bone density independent of increased energy intake. Although in one study[97] a particular calcium salt had some effect on bone mineral density when given to older women with very low calcium intake, there is no good evidence that increasing dietary calcium intake to > 500 mg/day in adults has any significant benefit. One trial[98] reported a reduction of lumbar spine bone loss after 1 year, but no subsequent reduction during a further 3 years of treatment. Calcium supplementation may prevent bone loss in older men and women[99], but there is no convincing evidence that calcium supplementation decreases the risk of fracture in patients with osteoporosis. It is very likely that any small increase in bone density achieved by alterations in dietary calcium intake is insufficient to prevent the rapid decrease that occurs in women around the time of the menopause. In summary, the evidence for increasing calcium intake to benefit the skeleton remains controversial[100]. However, given in conjunction with vitamin D, it probably has a useful role in the management of osteoporosis in the elderly[94].

LIFESTYLE CHANGES TO REDUCE BONE LOSS

All patients with osteoporosis and fractures should be given advice on lifestyle measures to decrease bone loss. These include eating a balanced diet rich in calcium, moderating tobacco and alcohol consumption, maintaining regular physical activity, and exposure to sunlight.

Exercise

In a previously sedentary patient, a program of regular exercise is not only likely to increase bone mineral density, but will probably also improve dexterity and muscle mass, thereby reducing the chances of serious fracture should a fall occur. Regular weight-bearing exercise produces a small benefit to bone density in postmenopausal women[101–103] but, by itself, is unable to prevent normal postmenopausal bone loss. One report[103] suggested that there may be a protective effect of lifelong and current exercise on hip bone mineral density in postmenopausal women, but no effect on fracture risk. It has been shown that the benefits gained by exercise are rapidly lost if a sedentary lifestyle is resumed[104]. Thus, exercise should be regarded as an adjuvant, rather than an alternative, to active treatment for osteoporosis.

Patients who are not osteoporotic should be encouraged to take up exercise that puts stress on weight-bearing bones, such as the spine or hip, as is appropriate to their cardiovascular fitness. Good examples are walking, jogging, and playing tennis. In established osteoporotics, exercise that involves jarring movements and flexion of the back should be avoided; the emphasis should be towards activity that encourages flexibility.

PREVENTION OF FALLS

Falls in the elderly are common, and occur more frequently in women and with advancing age[105]. Although it has been estimated that, in the general postmenopausal population, only 2–5% of falls result in fracture[106], and many of the predisposing factors are unavoidable (such as chronic ill health and cognitive impairment), strategies aimed at reducing avoidable risks may be expected to reduce the incidence of fracture. Such risks include the use of sedatives (including alcohol), wearing inappropriate footwear, hazardous home arrangements, and traveling in poor weather conditions.

There is some evidence that fall assessment is effective. A randomized controlled trial[107] in 301 elderly patients aged over 70 years, each with an apparent risk factor for falling, used assessment and modification of risk factors, and reported a reduction in falls to 35% over 12 months, compared with 47% in those receiving the usual healthcare

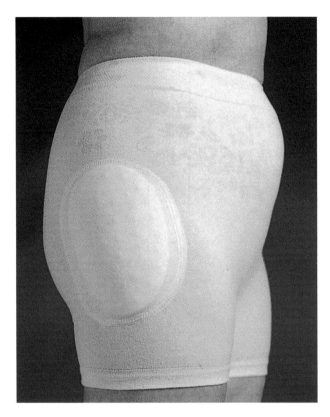

Figure 6.18 Hip protectors with rigid inserts have proved useful in preventing hip fracture in at-risk subjects. Courtesy of Robinson Healthcare, Chesterfield, UK

and social input. A British study[108] used similar methods in 397 community dwelling subjects aged over 65 years who had attended the emergency department with a fall. There was a significant 61% reduction in the risk of falls among the intervention group compared with the control group. Both studies were underpowered to detect a reduction in fracture incidence.

HIP PROTECTORS

An additional approach for reducing hip fracture is to prevent direct trauma to the hip with the use of hip protectors with rigid inserts (Figure 6.18). As the incidence of fracture following falls on the hip has been estimated to be much higher, approximately 24%, among nursing-home residents than in the general population, this group of subjects may benefit most from this form of treatment. In a study of nursing-home residents, Lauritzen and co-workers[109] showed that the relative

risk of hip fracture among women and men using hip protectors was 0.44 (95% CI 0.21–0.94). However, a recent meta-analysis of randomized and quasi-randomized trials[110] in which data from three individually randomized trials of 5135 community-dwelling participants were pooled, there was no reduction in hip fracture incidence with the provision of hip protectors (relative risk 1.16, CI 0.85–1.59). No evidence was found of any significant effect of hip protectors on the incidence of pelvic or other fractures. Compliance, particularly in the long term, was poor.

REFERENCES

1. Tuppurainen M, Kroger H, Honkanen R et al. Risks of perimenopausal fractures – a prospective population-based study. Acta Obstet Gynecol Scand 1995; 74: 624–8.

2. Paganini-Hill A, Ross RK, Gerkins VR et al. Menopausal estrogen therapy and hip fractures. Ann Intern Med 1981; 95: 28–31.

3. Weiss NS, Ure BL, Ballard JH et al. Decreased risk of fractures of the hip and lower forearm with postmenopausal use of estrogen. N Engl J Med 1980; 303: 1195–8.

4. Hutchinson TA, Polansky SM, Feinstein AR. Postmenopausal oestrogens protect against fractures of the hip and distal radius: a case-controlled study. Lancet 1979; 2: 705–9.

5. Ettinger B, Genant HK, Cann CE. Long term estrogen therapy prevents bone loss and fracture. Ann Intern Med 1979; 102: 319–24.

6. Baron YM, Brincat MP, Galea R, Calleja N. Intervertebral disc height in treated and untreated overweight menopausal women. Hum Reprod 2005; 20: 3566–70.

7. Lindsay R, Hart DM. The minimum effective dose of estrogen for prevention of postmenopausal bone loss. Obstet Gynecol 1984; 63: 759–63.

8. Christiansen C, Christensen MS, Larsen N-E, Transbol IB. Pathophysiological mechanisms of estrogen effect on bone metabolism. Dose–response relationships in early postmenopausal women. J Clin Endocrinol Metab 1982; 55: 1124–30.

9. Lees B, Stevenson JC. The prevention of osteoporosis using sequential low-dose hormone replacement therapy with estradiol-17β and dydrogesterone. Osteoporos Int 2001; 12: 251–8.

10. Rossouw JE, Anderson GL, Prentice RL et al. Writing Group for the Women's Health Initiative Investigators. Risks and benefits of estrogen plus progestin in healthy postmenopausal women: principal results from the Women's Health Initiative randomized controlled trial. JAMA 2002; 288: 321–33.

11. Anderson GL, Limacher M, Assaf AR et al. Women's Health Initiative Steering Committee. Effects of conjugated equine estrogen in postmenopausal women with hysterectomy: the Women's Health Initiative randomized controlled trial. JAMA 2004; 291: 1701–12.

12. McKay Hart D, Al-Azzawi F, Farish E. Effect of Ossopan alone, oestradiol implants alone or both therapies combined on bone density and bone biochemistry in oophorectomised women. In: Christiansen C, Johansen J, Riis BJ, eds. Osteoporosis. Copenhagen: Osteopress, 1987.

13. Ryde SJ, Bowen-Simkins K, Bowen-Simkins P et al. The effect of oestradiol implants on regional and total bone mass: a three-year longitudinal study. Clin Endocrinol 1994; 40: 33–8.

14. Savvas M, Watson NR, Garnett T et al. Skeletal effects of oral oestrogen compared with subcutaneous oestrogen and testosterone in postmenopausal women. BMJ 1988; 297: 331–3.

15. Holland EF, Leather AT, Studd JW. Increase in bone mass of older postmenopausal women with low mineral bone density after one year of percutaneous oestradiol implants. Br J Obstet Gynaecol 1995; 102: 238–42.

16. Riis BJ, Thomsen K, Strom V, Christiansen C. The effects of percutaneous estradiol and natural progesterone on postmenopausal bone loss. Am J Obstet Gynecol 1987; 156: 61–5.

17. Hillard TC, Whitcroft SJ, Marsh MS et al. Long-term effects of transdermal and oral hormone replacement therapy on postmenopausal bone loss. Osteoporos Int 1994; 4: 341–8.

18. Ettinger B, Genant HK, Cann CE. Postmenopausal bone loss is prevented by treatment with low dosage estrogen with calcium. Ann Intern Med 1987; 106: 40–5.

19. Lindsay D, Hart DM, Clark DM. Bone response to termination of oestrogen treatment. Lancet 1978; 1: 1325–7.

20. Wasnich RD, Bagger YZ, Hosking DJ et al. Early Postmenopausal Intervention Cohort Study Group. Changes in bone density and turnover after alendronate or estrogen withdrawal. Menopause 2004; 11: 622–30.

21. Stevenson JC, Kanis JA, Christiansen C. Bone-density measurement [Letter]. Lancet 1992; 339: 370–1.

22. Bagger YZ, Tankó LB, Alexandersen P et al. Two to three years of hormone replacement treatment in healthy women have long-term preventive effects on bone mass and osteoporotic fractures: the PERF study. Bone 2004; 34: 728–35.

23. Cauley JA, Seeley DG, Ensrud K et al. The Study of Osteoporotic Fractures Research Group. Estrogen replacement therapy and fractures in older women. Ann Intern Med 1995; 122: 9–16.

24. Kanis JA. Treatment of osteoporosis in elderly women. Am J Med 1995; 98: 60–6S.

25. Ettinger B, Ensrud KE, Wallace R et al. Effects of ultralow-dose transdermal estradiol on bone mineral density: a randomized clinical trial. Obstet Gynecol 2004; 104: 443–51.

26. Vedi S, Crocher PI, Garrahan NJ, Compston JE. Effects of hormone replacement therapy on cancellous bone structure in postmenopausal women. Bone 1996; 19: 69–72.

27. Stevenson JC. HRT, osteoporosis, and regulatory authorities. Quis custodiet ipsos custodies? Hum Reprod 2006; 21: 1668–71.

28. Torgerson DJ, Bell-Sayer SE. Hormone replacement therapy and prevention of vertebral fractures: a meta-analysis of randomized trials. BMC Musculoskelet Disord 2001; 2: 7.

29. Torgerson DJ, Bell-Sayer SE. Hormone replacement therapy and prevention of non-vertebral fractures: a meta-analysis of randomized trials. JAMA 2001; 285: 2891–7.

30. Delmas DD, Bjarnason NH, Mitlak BH et al. Effects of raloxifene on bone mineral density, serum cholesterol concentrations, and uterine endometrium in postmenopausal women. N Engl J Med 1997; 337: 1641–7.

31. Ettinger B, Black DM, Mitlak BH et al. Reduction of vertebral fracture risk in postmenopausal women with osteoporosis treated with raloxifene: results from a 3-year randomized clinical trial. Multiple Outcomes of Raloxifene Evaluation (MORE) Investigators. JAMA 1999; 282: 637–45.

32. Lippman ME, Kreuger KA, Eckert S et al. Indicators of lifetime estrogen exposure: effect on breast cancer incidence and interaction with raloxifene therapy in the multiple outcomes of raloxifene evaluation study patients. J Clin Oncol 2001; 19: 3111–16.

33. Barrett-Connor E, Mosca L, Collins P et al. Effects of raloxifene on cardiovascular events and breast cancer in postmenopausal women. N Engl J Med 2006; 355: 125–37.

34. Stevenson JC, ed. New Techniques in Metabolic Bone Disease. London: Wright, 1990: 63–8.

35. Gruber HE, Ivey JL, Baylink DJ et al. Long-term calcitonin therapy in postmenopausal osteoporosis. Metabolism 1984; 33: 295–303.

36. MacIntyre I, Stevenson JC, Whitehead MI et al. Calcitonin for the prevention of postmenopausal bone loss. Lancet 1988; 2: 1481–3.

37. Kollerup G, Hermann AP, Brixen K et al. Effects of salmon calcitonin suppositories on bone mass and turnover in established osteoporosis. Calcif Tissue Int 1994; 54: 12–15.

38. Reginster JY, Jupsin I, Deroisy R et al. Prevention of postmenopausal bone loss by rectal calcitonin. Calcif Tissue Int 1995; 56: 539–42.

39. Overgaard K, Riis BJ, Christiansen C et al. Nasal calcitonin the treatment of established osteoporosis. Clin Endocrinol 1989; 30: 435–42.

40. Reginster JY, Denis D, Albert A et al. 1-year controlled randomised trial of prevention of early postmenopausal bone loss by intranasal calcitonin. Lancet 1987; 2: 1481–3.

41. Overgaard K. Effect of intranasal salmon calcitonin therapy on bone mass and bone turnover in early postmenopausal women: a dose–response study. Calcif Tissue Int 1994; 55: 82–6.

42. Overgaard K, Lindsay R, Christiansen C. Patient responsiveness to calcitonin salmon nasal spray: a subanalysis of a 2-year study. Clin Ther 1995; 17: 680–5.

43. Reginster JY, Denis D, Deroisy R et al. Long-term (3 years) prevention of trabecular postmeno- pausal bone loss with low-dose intermittent nasal salmon calcitonin. J Bone Miner Res 1994; 9: 69–73.

44. Reginster JY, Deroisy R, Lecart MP et al. A dou- ble-blind, placebo-controlled, dose-finding trial of intermittent nasal salmon calcitonin for pre- vention of postmenopausal lumbar spine bone loss. Am J Med 1995; 98: 452–8.

45. Ellerington MC, Hillard TC, Whitcroft SI et al. Intranasal salmon calcitonin for the prevention and treatment of postmenopausal osteoporosis. Calcif Tissue Int 1996; 59: 6–11.

46. Silverman SL, Chesnut C, Andriano K et al. Salmon calcitonin nasal spray (NS-CT) reduces risk of vertebral fractures (VF) in established osteoporosis and has continuous efficacy with prolonged treatment: accrued worldwide data of the PROOF Study. Bone 1998; 23 (Suppl 5): 1108 (abstr).

47. Chestnut CH III, Silverman S, Andriano K et al. A randomised trial of nasal spray salmon calci- tonin in postmenopausal women with estab- lished osteoporosis: the prevent recurrence of osteoporotic fractures study. PROOF Study Group. Am J Med 2000; 109: 267–76.

48. Kanis JA, McCloskey EV. Effect of calcitonin on vertebral and other fractures. Q J Med 1999; 92: 143–9.

49. Lyritis GP, Paspati I, Karachalios T et al. Pain relief from salmon calcitonin in osteoporotic vertebral crush fractures. A double blind place- bo-controlled clinical study. Acta Orthop Scand 1997; 275: (Suppl): 112–14.

50. Storm T, Thamsborg G, Sorensen OH, Lund B. The effects of etidronate therapy in postmeno- pausal osteoporotic women: preliminary results. In: Christiansen C, Johansen J, Riis BJ, eds. Osteoporosis. Viborg: Norhaven Bogtrykken A/S, 1987: 1172–6.

51. Genant HK, Harris ST, Steiger P et al. The effects of etidronate therapy in postmenopausal osteoporotic women: preliminary results. In: Christiansen C, Johansen J, Riis BJ, eds. Osteoporosis. Viborg: Norhaven Bogtrykken A/S, 1987: 1177–81.

52. Roux C, Oriente P, Laan R et al. Randomized trial of effect of cyclical etidronate in the pre- vention of corticosteroid-induced bone loss. J Clin Endocrinol Metab 1998; 83: 1128–33.

53. van Staa TP, Abenhaim L, Cooper C. Use of cyclical etidronate and prevention of non-vertebral fractures. Br J Rheumatol 1998; 36: 1–8.

54. Valkema R, Papapoulis SE, Vismans F-JFE et al. A four-year continuous gain in bone mass in APD-treated osteoporosis. In: Christiansen C, Johansen J, Riis BJ, eds. Osteoporosis. Viborg: Norhaven Bogtrykken A/S, 1987: 836–9.

55. Reid IR, Wattie DJ, Evans MC et al. Continuous therapy with pamidronate, a potent bisphosphonate, in postmenopausal osteoporosis. J Clin Endocrinol Metab 1994; 79: 1595–9.

56. Lees B, Garland SW, Walton C et al. Role of oral pamidronate in preventing bone loss in postmenopausal women. Osteoporos Int 1996; 6: 480–5.

57. Liberman UA, Weiss SR, Broll J et al. The Alendronate Phase III Osteoporosis Treatment Study Group. Effect of oral alendronate on bone mineral density and the incidence of fractures in postmenopausal osteoporosis. N Engl J Med 1995; 333: 1437–43.

58. Chesnut CH IIIrd, McClung MR, Ensrud KE et al. Alendronate treatment of the postmenopausal osteoporotic woman: effect of multiple dosages on bone mass and bone remodeling. Am J Med 1995; 99: 144–52.

59. Black DM, Cummings SR, Karpf DB et al. The Fracture Intervention Trial Research Group. Randomised trial of effect of alendronate on risk of fracture in women with existing vertebral fractures. Lancet 1996; 348: 1535–41.

60. Harris ST, Watts NB, Genant HK et al. Effects of risedronate treatment on vertebral and non-vertebral fractures in women with postmenopausal osteoporosis: a randomized control trial. JAMA 1999; 282: 1344–52.

61. Reginster JY, Minne HW, Sorenson OH et al. Randomized trial of the effects of risedronate on vertebral fractures in women with established osteoporosis. Osteoporos Int 2000; 11: 83–91.

62. McClung MR, Geusens P, Miller PD et al. Effect of risedronate on the risk of hip fracture in elderly women. N Engl J Med 2001; 344: 333–40.

63. Epstein S. Ibandronate treatment for osteoporosis: rationale, preclinical, and clinical development of extended dosing regimens. Curr Osteoporos Rep 2006; 4: 14–20.

64. Dando TM, Noble S. Once-monthly ibandronate. Treat Endocrinol 2005; 4: 381–7; discussion 389–90.

65. Felsenberg D, Miller P, Armbrecht G et al. Oral ibandronate significantly reduces the risk of vertebral fractures of greater severity after 1, 2, and 3 years in postmenopausal women with osteoporosis. Bone 2005; 37: 651–4.

66. Emkey R, Koltun W, Beusterien K et al. Patient preference for once-monthly ibandronate versus once-weekly alendronate in a randomized, open-label, cross-over trial: the Boniva Alendronate Trial in Osteoporosis (BALTO). Curr Med Res Opin 2005; 21: 1895–903.

67. Reid IR, Brown JP, Burckhardt P et al. Intravenous zoledronic acid in postmenopausal women with low bone mineral density. N Engl J Med 2002; 346: 653–61.

68. Black DM, Delmas PD, Eastell R et al. Once yearly zoledronic acid for treatment of postmenopausal osteoporosis. N Engl J Med 2007; 356: 1809–22.

69. Marie PJ, Ammann P, Boivin G et al. Mechanisms of action and therapeutic potential of strontium in bone. Calcif Tissue Int 2001; 69: 121–9.

70. Meunier PJ, Roux C, Seeman E et al. The effects of strontium ranelate on the risk of vertebral fracture in women with postmenopausal osteoporosis. N Engl J Med 2004; 350: 459–68.

71. Reginster JY, Seeman E, De Vernejoul MC et al. Strontium ranelate reduces the risk of nonvertebral fractures in post-menopausal women with osteoporosis: Treatment of Peripheral Osteoporosis (TROPOS) study. J Clin Endocrinol Metab 2005; 90: 2816–22.

72. Kalu DN, Doyle FH, Pennock J, Foster GV. Parathyroid hormone and experimental osteosclerosis. Lancet 1970; 1: 1363–6.

73. Reeve J, Hesp R, Williams D et al. Anabolic effect of low doses of a fragment of human parathyroid hormone on the skeleton in postmenopausal osteoporosis. Lancet 1976; 1: 1035–8.

74. Reeve J, Meunier PJ, Parsons JA et al. Anabolic effect of human parathyroid hormone fragment on trabecular bone in involutional osteoporosis: a multicentre trial. BMJ 1980; 280: 1340–4.

75. Neer RM, Arnaud CD, Zanchetta AR et al. Effect of parathyroid hormone (1-34) on fractures and

bone mineral density in postmenopausal women with osteoporosis. N Engl J Med 2001; 344: 1434–41.

76. Lindsay R, Nieves J, Formica C et al. Randomised controlled study of effect of parathyroid hormone on vertebral-bone mass and fracture incidence among postmenopausal women on oestrogen with osteoporosis. Lancet 1997; 350: 550–5.

77. Body JJ, Gaich GA, Scheele WH et al. A randomized double-blind trial to compare the efficacy of teriparatide [recombinant human parathyroid hormone (1-34)] with alendronate in postmenopausal women with osteoporosis. J Clin Endocrinol Metab 2002; 87: 4528–35.

78. Dempster DW, Cosman F, Kurland EH et al. Effects of daily treatment with parathyroid hormone on bone microarchitecture and turnover in patients with osteoporosis: a paired biopsy study. J Bone Miner Res 2001; 16: 1846–53.

79. Jiang Y, Zhao JJ, Mitlak BH et al. Recombinant human parathyroid hormone (1-34) [teriparatide] improves both cortical and cancellous bone structure. J Bone Miner Res 2003; 18: 1932–41.

80. Black DM, Greenspan SL, Ensrud KE et al. The effects of parathyroid hormone alone or in combination in postmenopausal osteoporosis. N Engl J Med 2003; 349: 1207–15.

81. Finkelstein JS, Hayes A, Hunzelman JL et al. The effect of parathyroid hormone, alendronate, or both in men with osteoporosis. N Engl J Med 2003; 349: 1216–26.

82. Cosman F, Nieves J, Woelfert L et al. Alendronate does not block the anabolic effect of PTH in postmenopausal osteoporotic women. J Bone Miner Res 1998; 13: 1051–5.

83. Vahle JL, Long GG, Sandusky G et al. Bone neoplasms in F344 rats given teriparatide [rhPTH(1-34)] are dependent on duration of treatment and dose. Toxicol Pathol 2004; 32: 426–38.

84. Beneton MNC, Yates AJP, Rogers S et al. Stanozolol stimulates remodeling of trabecular bone and the net formation of bone at the endocortical surface. Clin Sci 1991; 81: 543–9.

85. Erdstieck RJ, Pols HA, van Kuijk C et al. Course of bone mass during and after hormone replacement therapy with and without addition of nandrolone decanoate. J Bone Miner Res 1994; 9: 277–83.

86. Mamelle N, Meunier PG, Dusan R et al. Risk–benefit ratio of sodium fluoride treatment in primary vertebral osteoporosis. Lancet 1988; 2: 361–5.

87. Riggs BL, Seeman E, Hodgson SF et al. Effect of the fluoride/calcium regimen on vertebral fracture occurrence in postmenopausal osteoporosis: comparison with conventional therapy. N Engl J Med 1982; 306: 446–50.

88. Baud CA, Very JM, Courvoisier B. Biophysical studies of bone mineral in biopsies of osteoporotic patients before and after long-term treatment with fluoride. Bone 1988; 9: 361–5.

89. Pak CY, Sakhaee K, Adams-Huet B et al. Treatment of postmenopausal osteoporosis with slow-release sodium fluoride. Final report of a randomized controlled trial. Ann Intern Med 1995; 123: 401–8.

90. Hedlund IR, Gallagher JC. Increased incidence of hip fracture in women treated with sodium fluoride. J Bone Miner Res 1989; 4: 223–5.

91. Ott SM, Chesnut CH. Calcitriol treatment is not effective in postmenopausal osteoporosis. Ann Intern Med 1989; 110: 267–74.

92. Nordin BEC, Horsman A, Crilly RG et al. Treatment of spinal osteoporosis in postmenopausal women. BMJ 1980; 280: 451–4.

93. Hansen MA. Assessment of age and risk factors on bone density and bone turnover in healthy premenopausal women. Osteoporos Int 1994; 4: 123–8.

94. Chapuy MC, Chapuy P, Thomas JL et al. Biochemical effects of calcium and vitamin D supplementation in elderly, institutionalized, vitamin D-deficient patients. Rev Rhum Mal Osteoartic (English edn) 1996; 63: 135–40.

95. Dawson-Hughes B, Harris SS, Krall EA et al. Rates of bone loss in postmenopausal women randomly assigned to one of two dosages of vitamin D. Am J Clin Nutr 1995; 61: 1140–5.

96. Lee PE, McElhaney JE, Dian L. Calcium and vitamin D supplementation for the prevention of fractures in postmenopausal women. Aging Health 2006; 2: 241–3.

97. Dawson-Hughes B, Dallal GE, Krall EA et al. A controlled trial of the effect of calcium supplementation on bone density in postmenopausal women. N Engl J Med 1990; 323: 878–83.

98. Reid IR, Ames RW, Evans MC et al. Long-term effects of calcium supplementation on bone loss and fractures in postmenopausal women: a randomized controlled trial. Am J Med 1995; 98: 331–5.

99. Peacock M, Liu G, Carey M et al. Effect of calcium or 25OH vitamin D3 dietary supplementation on bone loss at the hip in men and women over the age of 60. J Clin Endocrinol Metab 2000; 85: 3011–19.

100. Heaney RP. The role of nutrition in prevention and management of osteporosis. Clin Obstet Gynecol 1987; 50: 833–46.

101. Chow R, Harrison JE, Notarius C. Effects of two randomized exercise programmes on bone mass of healthy postmenopausal women. BMJ 1987; 295: 1441–4.

102. Lohman T, Going S, Pamenter R et al. Effects of resistance training on regional and total bone mineral density in premenopausal women: a randomized prospective study. J Bone Miner Res 1995; 10: 1015–24.

103. Greendale GA, Barrett-Connor E, Edelstein S et al. Lifetime leisure exercise and osteoporosis. The Rancho Bernardo study. Am J Epidemiol 1995; 14: 951–9.

104. Dalsky GP, Stocke KS, Ehsani AA et al. Weight-bearing exercise training and lumbar bone mineral content in postmenopausal women. Ann Intern Med 1988; 108: 824–8.

105. Prudham D, Evans JG. Factors associated with falls in the elderly: a community study. Age Ageing 1981; 10: 141–6.

106. Tinetti ME, Speechley M, Ginter SF. Risk factors for falls among elderly persons living in the community. N Engl J Med 1988; 319: 1701–7.

107. Tinetti ME, Baker DI, McAvay G et al. A multi-factorial intervention to reduce the risk of falling among elderly people living in the community. N Engl J Med 1994; 331: 821–7.

108. Close J, Ellis M, Hooper R et al. Prevention of falls in the elderly trial (PROFET): a randomised controlled trial. Lancet 1999; 353: 93–7.

109. Lauritzen JB, Petersen MM, Lund B. Effect of external hip protectors on hip fractures. Lancet 1993; 341: 11–13.

110. Parker MJ, Gillespie WJ, Gillespie LD. Effectiveness of hip protectors for preventing hip fractures in elderly people: systematic review. BMJ 2006; 332: 571–4.

CHAPTER 7

Conclusions

DIAGNOSIS AND SCREENING

Osteoporosis manifests itself clinically as fractures, but by the time the bone density has fallen to levels that predispose to fracture with minimal trauma, the treatment options have become more limited. Modern management aims to identify those patients who are at risk of developing fracture in the future.

Several studies have shown that the presence of risk factors in a given individual is not a good predictor of bone density[1–6]. Therefore, the risk of fracture must be predicted by measuring bone mineral density or identifying other factors that predispose to falls.

There have been no satisfactory studies of the effects of screening the whole population for osteoporosis. The role of risk factor assessment and different bone density techniques, frequency of screening, and identification of subgroups for which screening is most effective remain unclear[7].

It is unlikely that bone mineral density (BMD) screening of the early postmenopausal population will be valuable, as the BMD in the population at that time is quite high[8] and there is considerable individual variation in bone loss in the 10 years after the menopause. A screening program that utilizes hormone replacement therapy (HRT) as the treatment method is also unlikely to be successful, as long-term compliance with HRT is poor[9,10]. It remains to be established whether a screening program that uses dual-energy X-ray absorptiometry (DEXA) or ultrasound in the older postmenopausal population and that treats at-risk women with bisphosphonates or similar non-HRT treatment will be of value, but this form of program probably represents the most likely strategy for successful osteoporosis screening in the future.

In the absence of evidence for or against screening, our current policy for patients presenting at menopause clinics is to measure the bone mineral density using DEXA at the hip or spine in those women who present with osteoporotic fracture or risk factors for fracture.

TREATMENT

Estrogen replacement therapy is an appropriate method of treatment and prevention of osteoporosis and whose effects, both beneficial and adverse, have been widely studied. Although HRT use for the treatment of osteoporosis has declined as a result of patient concerns about breast cancer, and following the publication of studies that failed to show any overall effect of HRT on cardiovascular disease risk[11,12], HRT should remain a mainstay of treatment, particularly for prevention of the disease in younger postmenopausal women. It remains to be seen whether several years of therapy around the time of menopause can result in future fracture prevention for years to come.

Other current suitable treatments include bisphosphonates, selective estrogen receptor modulators (SERMs), strontium ranelate, and, in selected cases, teriparatide.

Patients with severe osteoporosis may benefit from the sequential use of one drug to stimulate bone formation followed by another to prevent resorption. The effectiveness of such combinations has not been studied extensively, and must be supervised by a physician who has experience of this method of treatment.

As it is likely that a small number of women will lose bone density while taking so-called standard bone-preserving treatments, it is advisable to repeat bone mineral density measurements in women who are known to have very low bone density before treatment. Unfortunately, the optimal management of the patient whose bone density falls while receiving standard monotherapy is unknown. Switching treatments or using combination therapies is a possible strategy.

The duration of therapy for the prevention or treatment of osteoporosis must be tailored to the needs of the given patient. Decisions concerning the duration of treatment may be guided by bone mineral density measurements. Thus, the patient who has been receiving HRT for 5 years and who wishes to stop therapy may need to start an alternative treatment such as a bisphosphonate if her bone mineral density estimation is significantly below that of her age-matched peers.

If bone density measurements are unavailable and general strategies of therapy must be adopted, then 5–10 years is generally considered to be the minimal duration of treatment necessary to significantly reduce the risk of fracture in at-risk populations. However, such general guidelines are a poor substitute for therapy that is determined by the requirements of the given individual.

Future therapies are likely to include the use of a monoclonal antibody to the RANKL (receptor activator of nuclear factor κB ligand; denosumab), which reduces bone resorption and increases bone density[13]. It is probable that new bisphosphonates will emerge. In addition, new forms of administration of parathyroid hormone (PTH) peptides are being developed[14]. Another form of HRT is under development, comprising the combination of estrogen with a SERM. This is hoped to produce the benefits of both compounds whilst avoiding some of their unwanted effects. Our options for the effective prevention and treatment of postmenopausal osteoporosis will continue to grow.

REFERENCES

1. Citron JT, Ettinger B, Genant HK. Prediction of peak premenopausal bone mass using a scale of weighted variables. In: Christiansen C, Johansesn J, Riis BJ, eds. Osteoporosis. Kobenhavn: Osteopress, 1987; 146–9.

2. Yano K, Wasnich RD, Vogel JM, Heilbrun LK. Bone mineral measurements among middle-aged and elderly Japanese residents in Hawaii. Ann J Epidemiol 1984; 119: 751–64.

3. Sowers MR, Wallace RD, Lemke JH. Correlates of mid-radius bone density among postmenopausal women: a community study. Am J Clin Nutr 1985; 41: 1045–53.

4. Kroger H, Tuppurainen M, Honkanen R et al. Bone mineral density and risk factors for osteoporosis – a population-based study of 1600 perimenopausal women. Calcif Tissue Int 1994; 55: 1–7.

5. Bauer DC, Browner WS, Cauley JA et al. The Study of Osteoporosis Fractures Research Group. Factors associated with appendicular bone mass in older women. Ann Intern Med 1993; 118: 657–65.

6. Wasnich RD, Ross PD, Vogel JM, Maclean CJ. The relative strengths of osteoporotic risk factors in a prospective study of postmenopausal osteoporosis. J Bone Miner Res 1987; 2 (Suppl 1): 343.

7. Nelson HD, Helfand M, Woolf SH, Allan JD. Screening for postmenopausal osteoporosis: a review of the evidence for the US Preventive Services Task Force [see comment]. Ann Intern Med 2002; 137: 529–41.

8. Pesonen J, Sirola J, Tuppurainen M et al. High bone mineral density among perimenopausal women. Osteoporos Int 2005; 16: 1899–906.

9. Ravnikar A. Compliance with hormone therapy. Am J Obstet Gynecol 1987; 156: 1332–4.

10. Wallace WA, Price VA, Elliot CA et al. Hormone replacement therapy: acceptability to Nottingham postmenopausal women with a risk factor for osteoporosis. J R Soc Med 1990; 83: 699–701.

11. Rossouw JE, Anderson GL, Prentice RL et al. Writing Group for the Women's Health Initiative Investigators. Risks and benefits of estrogen plus progestin in healthy postmenopausal women: principal results from the Women's Health Initiative randomized controlled trial. JAMA 2002; 288: 321–33.

12. Anderson GL, Limacher M, Assaf AR et al. Women's Health Initiative Steering Committee. Effects of conjugated equine estrogen in post-menopausal women with hysterectomy: the Women's Health Initiative randomized controlled trial. JAMA 2004; 291: 1701–12.

13. McClung MR, Lewiecki EM, Cohen SB et al. Denosumab in postmenopausal women with low bone mineral density. N Engl J Med 2006; 354: 821–31.

14. Sato K. Therapeutic agents for disorders of bone and calcium metabolism. Development of nasal formulation of hPTH (1-34). Clin Calcium 2007; 17: 64–71.

Index

Page numbers in *italic* denote material in Figures or Tables.

OBSTETRICS AND GYNAECOLOGY/ REPRODUCTIVE MEDICINE

Informa Healthcare provides a wide range of Obstetrics and Gynaecology journals.

Journal of Obstetrics and Gynaecology

Journal of Obstetrics and Gynaecology represents an established forum for the entire field of obstetrics and gynaecology with an affiliation with the British Society for the Study of Vulval Disease (BSSVD). It publishes a broad range of high quality original, peer-reviewed papers, from scientific and clinical research to reviews relevant to practice and case reports.

www.informaworld.com/cjog

Editors in Chief: Harry Gordon, Alan MacLean

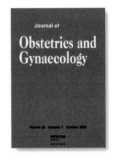

Climacteric

Climacteric is the official Journal of the International Menopause Society with a current Impact Factor of 2.299, ranking it in the top tier of all journals in obstetrics and gynaecology. It has an increased frequency of 6 issues per year.

www.informaworld.com/dcli

Editor in Chiefs: David Sturdee, Alastair MacLennan

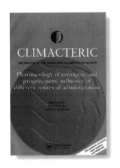

The Journal of Maternal-Fetal and Neonatal Medicine

This monthly publication is the official journal of the European Association of Perinatal Medicine, the Federation of Asia and Oceania Perinatal Societies, and the International Society of Perinatal Obstetricians. It publishes a wide range of peer-reviewed original research on the obstetric, medical, genetic, mental health and surgical complications of pregnancy and their effects on the mother, fetus and neonate.

www.informaworld.com/djmf

Editors in Chief: Gian Carlo Di Renzo, Dev Maulik

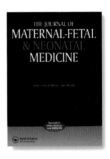

The European Journal of Contraception and Reproductive Health Care

For over 11 years, *The European Journal of Contraception and Reproductive Health Care* is the official journal of the European Society of Contraception. It has published published original peer-reviewed research papers, review papers and other appropriate educational material on all aspects of contraception and reproductive health care.

www.informaworld.com/dejc

Editor in Chief: Jean-Jacques Amy,

Editors: Medard Lech, Dan Apter, Dimitris Lazaris

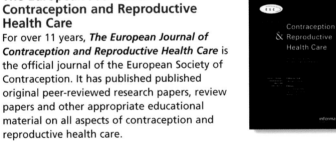

Journal of Psychosomatic Obstetrics and Gynecology

Journal of Psychosomatic Obstetrics and Gynecology is the official journal of the International Society of Psychosomatic Obstetrics and Gynecology. It provides a scientific forum for gynaecologists, psychiatrists and psychologists as well as for all those who are interested in the psychosocial and psychosomatic aspects of women's health.

www.informaworld.com/dpog

Editors in Chief: Willibrord C.M Weijmar Schultz, Harry B.M Van de Wiel

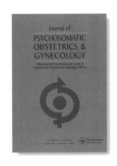

Gynecological Endocrinology

Gynecological Endocrinology, published monthly is the official journal of the International Society of Gynecological Endocrinology. It includes topics relating to the control and function of the different endocrine glands in females, the effects of reproductive events on the endocrine System and the consequences of endocrine disorders on reproduction.

www.informaworld.com/dgye

Editor in Chief: Andrea R. Genazzani

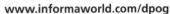

Human Fertility

Human Fertility is the official Journal of the British Fertility Society, the Association of Clinical Embryologists, the British Infertility Counselling Association, the Royal College of Nursing Fertility Nurses Group, and the British Andrology Society. Topics include molecular medicine and healthcare delivery.

www.informaworld.com/thuf

Editor in Chief: Henry Leese

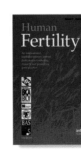

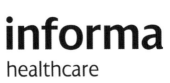

Only £45/AU$110

Pathology

Special theme issue: Gynaecological pathology
Invited guest editor: Peter Russell

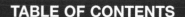

TABLE OF CONTENTS

This special theme issue on Gynaecological Pathology contains contributions from some of the finest international pathologists in the field. They provide an insight into common yet difficult aspects of surgical pathology of the female reproductive tract.

Visit **www.informaworld.com/pathology**
for general Journal information

To order the special issue, contact:
Louise Porter, Marketing Manager, Informa Healthcare,
69-77 Paul Street, London, EC2A 4LQ; **Email:** Louise.Porter@informa.com

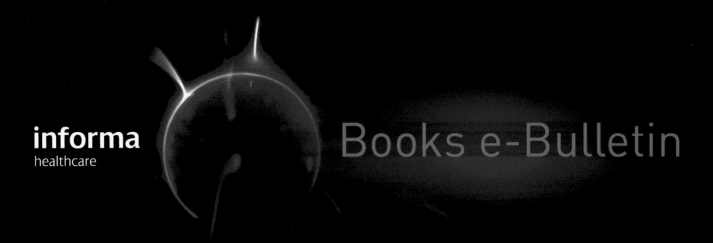
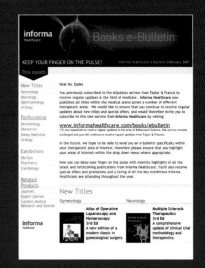